2030: The Future of Medicine

About Richard

Richard has spent most of his career in healthcare, as a leader of organizations, as a board member and as a consultant. His leadership roles have spanned therapeutics, diagnostics and informatics, both in the United States and in Europe. He was recently voted as one of the top 50 most influential people in UK healthcare and he sits on several healthcare and life sciences advisory boards on both sides of the Atlantic.

His passions include securing a sustainable future for healthcare and redesigning how new medical technology is brought into practice. He now lives in London but is a frequent visitor to the US, where he spent 11 years working in Boston, New Haven, New York, and San Francisco.

"A very engaging and enjoyable read, covering a colossal amount of ground without feeling stretched... translating the more upstream science into practical implications for the general public. A great primer on the health future—for both the health-informed and those coming to such thoughts for the first time."

Sam Lister, Health Editor, the *London Times*

"The next 20 years will see huge strides in how medical science could transform our lives. This book not only describes what will be possible but also whether and how we can afford it."

Professor George Poste, Del E. Webb Chair in
Health Innovation, Arizona State University

"An accessible and comprehensive snapshot of the complex healthcare environment with which policy makers wrestle...laying out the tremendous tensions that exist in a manner which leaves a sense of optimism not defeat. A must read for those who want to be part of solutions to get best treatments to the most people and allow us all to benefit from one of the most remarkably exciting fields of human activity...understanding and fixing ourselves."

Andrew Witty, Chief Executive, GlaxoSmithKline

"This book is a must for healthcare leaders on both sides of the Atlantic. It grapples with the big question of how we can afford the future."

Ken Jennings, Consultant to leading US health systems
and author of best-selling book *The Servant Leader*.

2030: The Future of Medicine

Avoiding a Medical Meltdown

Dr Richard Barker, MA, FRSM

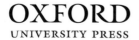

OXFORD
UNIVERSITY PRESS

OXFORD
UNIVERSITY PRESS

Great Clarendon Street, Oxford OX2 6DP

Oxford University Press is a department of the University of Oxford.
It furthers the University's objective of excellence in research, scholarship,
and education by publishing worldwide In

Oxford New York

Auckland Cape Town Dar es Salaam Hong Kong Karachi
Kuala Lumpur Madrid Melbourne Mexico City Nairobi
New Delhi Shanghai Taipei Toronto

With offices in

Argentina Austria Brazil Chile Czech Republic France Greece
Guatemala Hungary Italy Japan Poland Portugal Singapore
South Korea Switzerland Thailand Turkey Ukraine Vietnam

Oxford is a registered trade mark of Oxford University Press
in the UK and in certain other countries

Published in the United States
by Oxford University Press Inc., New York

British Library Cataloguing in Publication Data
Data available

Library of Congress Cataloging in Publication Data
Data available

Typeset by Newgen Imaging Systems (P) Ltd., Chennai, India
Printed in Great Britain
on acid-free paper by
Ashford Colour Press Ltd., Gosport, Hampshire

ISBN 978-0-19-960066-3

10 9 8 7 6 5 4 3 2 1

Contents

Acknowledgements

I owe a great debt to many close colleagues over the years, in the diverse British and American organizations serving the world of healthcare for which it has been my privilege to work. Colleagues from McKinsey, IBM, Chiron, iKnowMed, Molecular Staging, the ABPI, and the NHS will all recognize insights gained while working together in these very different settings.

However, those who kindly read, critiqued, and improved this book deserve particular thanks: Professors Adrian Towse and Nancy Devlin of the Office of Health Economics; Professor Sir Alasdair Breckenridge, Chairman of the UK Medicines and Healthcare Products Regulatory Agency (MHRA); Professor Sir Michael Rawlins, Chairman of the National Institute for Health and Clinical Excellence (NICE); Professor Nick Bosanquet of Imperial College; Sam Lister, Health Editor of the London Times. All commented very helpfully.

Thanks, too, to my editor at Oxford University Press, Nic Wilson, who has been unfailingly encouraging and helpful from the outset.

Any errors and omissions are mine alone, of course.

My thanks go also to my wife Michaela, who has been both inspiring and tolerant as this book took shape. I'm also grateful for three wonderful children, Daniel, Joseph, and Hannah, for their encouragement and love over the years.

It is to their children that the book is dedicated: they will inherit the healthcare innovations we see by 2030, and the changes we make to the healthcare system in the intervening years. My hope is that these changes will be for the better.

Abbreviations

ABPI	Association of the British Pharmaceutical Industry
AIDS	acquired immunodeficiency syndrome
ARP	Alzheimer's risk profile
AVM	arteriovenous malformation
BMI	body mass index
CME	continuing medical education
COMT	catechol O-methyl transferase
COPD	chronic obstructive pulmonary disease
CT	computerized tomography
DNA	deoxyribonucleic acid
DRG	diagnostic-related groups
EMR	electronic medical record
ESC	embryonic stem cell
FDA	Food and Drug Administration
GCP	good clinical practice
GDP	gross domestic product
GINA	Genetic Non-discrimination Act
GP	General Practitioner
HDL	high-density lipoprotein
HIV	human immunodeficiency virus
HMO	Health Maintenance Organization
HTA	health technology assessment
IBS	irritable bowel syndrome
IHS	integrated health systems
IQWG	Institute for Quality and Efficiency in Health Care
LDL	low-density lipoprotein
MBP	myelin basic protein
MHRA	Medicines and Healthcare Products Regulatory Agency
MN	motor neuron disease

MRI	magnetic resonance imaging
MRSA	methicillin-resistant Staphylococcus aureus
NHS	National Health Service
NICE	National Institute for Health and Clinical Excellence
OECD	Organisation for Economic Co-operation and Development
PBR	payment by results
PCT	Primary Care Trust
PDP	product development partnerships
PEPFAR	President's Emergency Plan for AIDS Relief
PET	positron emission tomography
QALY	quality-adjusted life year
QOF	Quality and Outcomes Framework
RSV	respiratory syncytial virus
SAE	serious adverse events
SAEC	Serious Adverse Events Consortium
SC4SM	Stem Cells for Safer Medicines
siRNA	small interfering RNA molecules
SNP	Single Nucleotide Polymorphisms
SPARCS	See-Plan-Act-Refine-Communicate
SSRI	selective serotonin reuptake inhibitors
TNF	tumour necrosis factor

Introduction and summary

Sometimes our future is hidden in plain sight. This is true of the future of our healthcare, as explored in this book—written for all those involved in healthcare, practitioners and patients, who want to know what awaits them.

Over the last couple of years, the credit crunch has driven a near-collapse of the world's financial systems. With the benefit of hindsight, many say this could have been avoided. But it all seemed to happen so fast. Much of the prosperity of the last two decades was built on unaffordable levels of debt, debt that had built up over years, yet could bankrupt seemingly impregnable banks overnight. Everyone asked: how did we not see this meltdown coming? Could we have done anything to head it off?

Over the next 10–20 years, I believe healthcare is headed for its own meltdown. The warning signs are there, the crisis is already being predicted, but unlike the financial meltdown it will unfold over years, not weeks and months. We still have time to avoid it, if we act now. So this book is written for all those who care about the future of medicine: particularly in the two nations in which I have spent most of my career—the US and the UK—but also in those countries that share similar problems, or want to avoid them as their systems develop. I hope enough non-specialists will read it for it to trigger debate beyond the medical world, since the future of medicine is too important to be left to experts.

In the US, the air has been full of debates on healthcare reform—ObamaCare—aiming to give health coverage to millions without it. Welcome as this development is, it will add billions of dollars in cost to an already incredibly expensive system. In Britain, the home of universal coverage since 1948, the controversies are different, but not the underlying concerns about affordability. The arguments surrounding the National Health Service (NHS) are how to free it from political influence, how to get the most healthcare for the pound, and whether national targets or local control delivers better outcomes. In both countries total health costs rise faster than the rest of the economy, and look likely to do so as far as the eye can see, without draconian cutbacks.

Real solutions to avoid 'medical meltdown' on either side of the Atlantic must get to the heart of the dual problem in healthcare—ever-growing supply *and* escalating demand. This book offers a penetrating analysis of this underlying problem, and offers some clear, but far-reaching solutions.

The author is a bioscientist who has spent most of his working life in and around medicine. So I start with how discoveries in bioscience will revolutionize medicine over the coming decades. But the central issue in healthcare over the next 20 years is not the onward march of medical science. It is the collision of these new and often expensive possibilities with our ever-growing demand for healthcare of all kinds, today's as well as tomorrow's. Can we afford all the care we'd like to have *and* all the new medicines and procedures under development?

The **supply** of new medical technology, described in Chapter 1, exploits the huge advances we are making in bioscience. We are building up a profound understanding of how the beautiful molecular machines of the living cell actually work, and how they link together in the almost unimaginably complex system that is our body. As the pace of biological advance quickens, it poses several major questions. Over the next 20 years, what fresh pharmaceutical innovations are on the horizon? Will gene and cell therapy reach the diseases that drugs cannot reach? 'Personalized medicine', ensuring a patient receives only the care that works for them, sounds ideal, but is it practical? Different technologies are converging—therapeutics, diagnostics, informatics, nanotechnology: what will they bring us? Intelligent, miniaturized devices implanted in us, to sense impending disease and deliver therapy automatically?

The power of healthcare information is transforming the healthcare landscape. The day of comprehensive, portable electronic medical records is dawning: will they usher in a revolution in how care is planned, delivered, and tailored to the individual? Will health systems start to learn from experience? Medical images are gaining in quality and power. From the beautiful intricacy of the human body revealed by Galen's dissections, it has taken mankind many centuries to move from dissection of the dead to the tools that reveal the inner workings of the living. How will this new power change medicine?

Technical wizardry puts new power at the fingertips of the medical profession, but they face some powerful challenges from other directions. Better informed patients, more cost-conscious payers, and the ever-present threat of legal liability, makes doctoring an increasingly complex affair. The old omniscient, priestly role is being replaced by that of a specialized technical advisor, whose actions are hedged around by guidelines, formularies and approval systems. How will the role of medics and the structure of medical care change?

In Chapter 2 we turn to the **demand** for healthcare, and the combined impact of ageing, of new disease threats, and ever-heightened expectations about health. Mankind's expectations of a healthy, vigorous lifespan have increased dramatically. Longer lifespan is clearly good news, but age brings with it intensified health needs—treatments for cancer, for neurodegenerative diseases like Alzheimer's, and for the repair and restoration of the body from longer years of wear and tear.

However, much of the future demand for health services seems destined to come from self-inflicted disease—from obesity, diabetes, alcohol-associated disease, and that reliable killer, smoking. The long-term consequences of these diseases for the health of nations and the cost of healthcare are enormous.

While improved public health and better treatment have rolled back many diseases, nature has a rich supply of new challenges—in the form of pandemics of infectious disease jumping from other species to mankind, and then spreading rapidly across an ever more interconnected world.

Partly as a result of such pandemics, global healthcare's greatest demands are in the world's least developed countries. Despite the rhetoric of world leaders, and new funding from philanthropists, progress is pitiful in too many countries. Both for humanitarian reasons, and out of naked self-interest, we must find ways for the triumphs of medicine to reach the poorest parts of the world.

All health systems are already groaning as they grapple with today's funding limitations with today's medical technology. Patient co-payments, treatment rationing, budgetary controls – all are symptoms of the pressure to make ends meet. The US is heading for 20% of its GDP spent on healthcare, and other advanced economies are moving in the same direction. The healthcare bill is rising faster than our ability to raise taxes, or insurance premiums.

The effect of the supply and demand forces driving up health care costs is illustrated in Figure A1.

So, the third chapter tackles the changes urgently needed if **meltdown** is to be avoided. Ten radical healthcare levers can make the vital difference between balance and bankruptcy. But they have to be pulled soon, and pulled together.

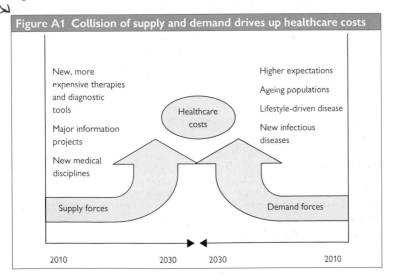

Figure A1 Collision of supply and demand drives up healthcare costs

New, more expensive therapies and diagnostic tools

Major information projects

New medical disciplines

Supply forces

Healthcare costs

Higher expectations

Ageing populations

Lifestyle-driven disease

New infectious diseases

Demand forces

2010   2030   2030   2010

The 10 changes sound deceptively simple, but made together their impact on healthcare, medical practice, the experience of patients and the affordability of the outcomes would be profound.

The costs of healthcare supply can be transformed by the personalization of care, by an end-to-end approach to chronic disease and by redesigning care delivery to bring it closer to the home and the community. The costs of new technology must also be radically reduced, by streamlining its development and managing its risks more intelligently.

The costs driven by demand can also be radically reduced. Prevention strategies are vital but must be based less on public health campaigns and more on personal health management, with patients empowered as never before, to manage their diet, weight, and exercise and to take prompt action when symptoms appear. Hard choices are needed on what treatments to offer, but these should be made on the basis of value, assessed by outcomes achieved, not just cost. To improve both outcomes and costs, incentives for professionals and for patients must be properly aligned, giving positive financial reasons to deliver, and receive, efficient care.

Two other levers can affect both supply and demand. The first is our attitude to waste: elimination of ineffective care, inefficient patient pathways, and outmoded medical practice. But the most powerful lever of all is integrated patient care based on integrated information. If information about past care, options for future care, and all the factors to guide these choices, could be brought together around the patient, this would unlock the full potential of the other nine levers.

Chapter 4, an **agenda for change**, deals with how the levers should be pulled. When faced with a major problem too often we say: 'they' must do this and that, meaning politicians and policymakers. But all of us—professionals, suppliers, care managers, and patients—have vital roles to play in creating the momentum for change.

Yes, there is a role for governments. With healthcare perhaps the highest profile, longest-running of political issues, there is a demanding policy agenda for the next 20 years. But first we need a mindset change, a new synthesis between health and economic policy. Most investment in health and in health technologies should not be seen as an economic burden but as an enabler of economic growth. However, responsibility does not end with politicians—indeed their detailed meddling with health management can cause more problems than it solves. The managers and users of the health system must also shoulder responsibility for avoiding the meltdown. The way in which care is designed and delivered, the habits of the well and the self-management of patients all have to change radically.

Finally, in a short fifth chapter of conclusions, we reflect on the very different problems and challenges of the two systems on which this book focuses most—the US and the UK. What can they learn from each other? Is there a way forward that combines the best of both?

So this is not a book of theory, but an agenda for practical action. It paints a picture of the future in order to urge action now. We will use the everyday life of a family in 2030 to illustrate what is possible if we succeed. As we map supply, demand and their future collision we will view the questions, choices and challenges of the future of medicine through their eyes. Meet the Carter family.

The Carter Family

Jane is 56, and she sits at her desk at home, staring thoughtfully into the middle distance, her morning coffee cooling, unnoticed. No-one to disturb her reverie. Her children **Susannah**, **Caroline**, and **Keith** are grown, and not just grown …. the birth last year, to Susannah and husband Maurice, of little **Bernie**, the apple of her eye, has just ushered in the next generation. So soon! So she feels just a little old, yet fully and gloriously young, all at the same time. Once, she muses, hers would have been called the sandwich generation, with parents and children to worry about simultaneously. Now it's perfectly normal to have three generations to parent, all at once!

Not that her mother and father are exactly in their dotage: he still has an iron grip—on your hand, on his woodworking tools, and on the world around him. And she still has her grip on him, poor fellow. It is January 1, 2030, and the morning mist has lifted to reveal a sharp and clear start to the New Year. Like most mothers, she focuses her new year's resolutions not on herself but on those around her.

George, her husband …. he's OK, but thinking with a small smile of his now receding hairline she wants to stave off the ravages of time as long as possible—for all sorts of reasons. So let's start with his health profile. His total cancer scan last year revealed not even the beginnings of abnormality anywhere, she was relieved to see. But the cardiovascular markers confirmed what he had known for 10 years now—with his genes, only a tough lifelong diet and his individual regimen of lipid reducers and immuno-modulators would safeguard his heart for the next 40 years. The latest cardiopredictor gave it only 35, unless he got back into the gym—and stayed out of the bakery so temptingly placed on his way home.

So her first resolution is to bring that number back up to forty by the end of the year. What of her **Susannah**, her daughter? She probably won't need to worry there yet: before Bernie was born, Susannah and **Maurice** went through all the genetic profiling available, just to be sure. So she knew to be careful with her blood pressure and calcium in pregnancy, and now knows that her bones will stay strong for many years yet if she just has one slow-release capsule a week with the right mix of minerals and

(Continued)

medicines. And keeps up her twice-a-week tennis. The health plan individually designed for the family, taking into account all that was found, now makes compliance with the family's medical regimens a matter of money, not just virtue. If they skip their health screens, medicines or exercise their premium rises. But at least that focuses the mind!

The phone rings, piercing her reverie. It's her mother-in-law, **Rose**. And her voice is troubled. **Phil**, her husband, 82, has awoken with numbness down one side of his body. It's not unusual, she can't help thinking, for his occasional over-indulgence to leave him groggy in the morning, but this sounds different. Should she drive him to hospital? Can she come over? Should he stay in bed? The questions tumble out. Most importantly, says Jane, make sure his health monitor is plugged in and transmitting blood pressure, pulse, glucose, and other vital signs to the LiveCheck service. Ever since he became diabetic, this service has been literally a lifeline for them. Now it can transmit to the hospital all the key information on how this problem developed. Hurriedly, Jane wakes her husband and together they decide to drive over...

The 21st century has ushered in a host of challenges—global warming, energy and water shortages, societal stress—these will all be issues for the Carter family. But the issue that touches them and all of us, from presidents to paupers, most closely is healthcare. Its supply and demand are on a collision course—and unless we can avert the resulting meltdown in healthcare over the next 20 years, we and the Carters will see rationing, growing inequality, needless suffering and in some cases premature death. This book is about creating a different future: one for Jane, her family, and for the rest of us. An affordable and sustainable one.

Chapter 1

The supply of new
medicine—unlimited?

Medical advance is still in the foothills of its potential. Past centuries gave us herbal remedies, leeches, poultices, surgery, anaesthetics and other basic tools, but it is just in the last 50 years that we have seen precise, knowledge-based intervention in the processes of disease. And only in the last 20 that our burgeoning knowledge of bioscience has enabled us to design drugs with their molecular target specifically in view.

Medicines have been discovered to combat ulcers, control the high blood pressure and cholesterol that trigger strokes and heart attacks, halt the invasion of HIV, and arrest the progress of arthritis and of cancer. We have developed powerful, penetrative and precise body scanning technologies to identify and map disease, and track its treatment. We have seen the emergence of 'keyhole' surgery. We have created transplant and implant solutions, both for catastrophic failures of organs and the erosion of joints.

In his book *The Rise and Fall of Modern Medicine*, James Le Fanu asserted that in future we will not see this pace of progress sustained. I beg to differ. The pace of progress will not just continue, it will accelerate. There are at least eight frontiers on which we are poised to make further huge advances in knowledge and in practice: (1) a new deeper understanding of how our biology is wired together, (2) further advances in drug therapy, based on these new insights, (3) the implantation of genes and cells to regenerate bodily function, (4) the exciting visualization of biology in action, by new imaging techniques, (5) tools that move us closer to the ideal of 'personalized medicine', (6) integrated health information, long-promised but finally delivering, (7) smart devices that combine bioengineering with intelligence, (8) the implications of all these for medical practitioners, with advanced therapies, accelerating specialism, and expert systems revolutionizing their working lives.

Bioscience—a new age of 'systems' understanding

Since the genomic age dawned just over half a century ago, almost every day has brought new insights into how life works. But we are still just scratching the surface. In the hundreds of millions of years from the first self-replicating fragment of life to today's vast variety of life-forms, biology has developed staggering complexity.

We know the DNA sequence of the 30,000 genes in the human genome. It is like a massive computer program, the meaning of which we are only beginning to glimpse. However, this program does not alone fix the final outcome: identical twins (with identical gene sequences) still have different fingerprints. So even in our earliest days, a single genetic message can have different results. We still have a great deal to discover about how the genetic program becomes the organism in all its complexity.

We now know in some detail how DNA is copied, how it is translated into the proteins making up the cellular machinery, and how some of these proteins play their role in the molecular dance of the cell, but there the clarity ends. The complex process by which genes are switched on and off, the patterns of interaction between the 150,000 or so proteins that are encoded by our genes, the ways in which each cell 'knows' what it is and what tasks it should perform—these are the questions that now occupy bioscientists.

We have a name for this staggering complexity—systems biology. For life is indeed a system, a massive wiring diagram or metro map, one with 30,000 genes, 150,000 proteins and hundreds of chemical messengers (metabolites) all of which can, in principle, affect all the others.

It is the total system, not the genetic programme alone, that makes us what we are. Humans share 98% of their genetic message with chimpanzees, nearly half with the humble fruit fly, and even a third with the simplest of worms. So we can see that it is less the content of the code and more how the messages flow and interact that defines us.

Unravelling this complexity, the metro map of life, will be the work of the next hundred years. But we are already mapping some of the biochemical pathways that are critical both when they work, in health, and when they don't, in disease.

Sometimes a disease has a simple origin—a single gene mutation that results in a protein that fails to function as it should. Such genetic disorders, passed through generations, may have minor, or quite devastating health consequences. In some cases the biochemical discovery leads us straight to the treatment. The lack of key metabolic enzymes cuts short human lives while still in their teens, or even earlier. But with products such as Cerizyme, which replaces a fat-digesting enzyme lacked by sufferers from Gaucher's disease, these conditions can now be treated, and much longer lives result.

The majority of diseases, however, are 'multigenic'—that is, they result from disorders across many genes and pathways. And individuals vary in how these pathways function, because of subtle differences in their gene sequences—so-called Single Nucleotide Polymorphisms (SNPs).

Just a single letter SNP change can have huge consequences—either in how the gene behaves or in the way the protein it codes for operates. The fruit fly has just one mutation that, when present, turns it from a two-wing to a four-wing version—in effect turning evolution back on itself.

Single-site changes to the human gene sequence can change the structure of a protein, and so increase or decrease how well a medicine binds to it, resulting in greater (or weaker) effectiveness of the therapy. The small SNP differences between individuals' sequences occur in about one DNA letter in 500—but this means 6 million gene differences between two people!

These large numbers have driven a new era of 'high throughput' biology. We now have technology for SNP counting that can achieve a rate of 4 million a day. So individual gene profiles that what would have taken literally years to do can now be done in a matter of hours.

The effects of interfering with a specific protein ripple through the rest of the cell's pathways. Despite the goal of designing a drug to do only one job in one location, it binds and affects the biology in others. As a result, many drugs, however carefully designed, have minor, or sometimes serious side-effects, and this determines the benefit versus risk of the drug.

The tools we now have to study these 'ripple' effects are bringing fascinating insights. Scientists use chips that show the pattern of gene expression (which genes are turned on to produce proteins)—for example in the liver, vital for eliminating drugs from the body when they have done their work.

Applying gene expression chips to cancerous tumours has shown the extraordinary diversity of gene expression between patients that formerly seemed to have the same disease. This helps to tune drug regimens to different tumour types. We have also discovered that cancer's course can be changed by the genes that are activated to defend against it. No less than 500 genes are themselves changed by diet and exercise, giving the basis for self-help regimes to assist the battle against disease.

The greatest insights will come from determining the full genome sequence of not just one, but millions of individuals. Already the rate of gene sequencing has been multiplied, and its costs reduced by more than a thousand-fold. One of the landmarks that scientists are using is the '$1,000 genome'—a complete sequence for less than a thousand dollars. This landmark is now within reach.

The same rapid advances are being made in all the downstream steps of the biological cascade—gene expression, protein concentration, cell analysis, and so on. These powerful tools are turning biology from a science of observation to one of information processing. As Lee Hood, founder of the Institute of Systems Biology in Seattle puts it: 'systems biology is information science'. In the Institute, biological scientists mingle with information scientists, determining the impact of variations in genes, their expression and the level and type of proteins they produce and feeding them into ever-more sophisticated computer models of the pathways and control mechanisms of the cell.

Can we glimpse what new avenues of medical advance might open up from these new 'systems' insights? Two examples. First, if we can fully understand the differences between the proteins on the surface of cancer cells and their normal cousins, we may be able to selectively activate macrophages (killer cells in the body's immune system) to recognize and destroy the cancer—a task they already perform but which some cancer cells still escape.

A second is more far-reaching, but already visible on the horizon. If we can fully determine all human genetic polymorphisms and their health significance, a complete gene sequence of an individual will give us their 'future health history', to use Dr Hood's phrase. Then if we can study, at regular points on the person's lifespan, the expression of those genes and the profile of proteins they produce, this will give us an instant read-out of where the individual is in their molecular life history. An early warning of future disease, before any symptoms appear.

'Systems' insights need not stop at the level of the machinery inside the cell. The whole organism is the result of the interaction between cells, and the behaviour of an individual cell reflects the signals it receives from others around it.

Exciting new avenues are opening up in the fight against cancer beyond the specific targeting of genes and proteins in the cancerous cell, to focus on the environment around it. As one cancer researcher has said: 'cancer is no more a disease of the cell than a traffic jam is a problem of the individual car'. So cancer can be viewed as a disease of cellular organization. If cancerous cells are placed in a different environment, such as in an embryo, they can revert to normal function. Understanding and then interfering with this signalling between cancer cells and the normal cells around them could restrain or even reverse the spread of cancer.

So, as a result of all these basic science advances, what insights might we have in 20 years that are not yet available to medicine? New, more precise medicines that interact with the body's biological networks in more sophisticated and predictable ways. Chips to recognize genetic traits from just a drop of blood. Urine tests that tell us if cancer is emerging. Tools to show us when a protein does not fold as it should, and starts to stick together to form damaging deposits in the brain, as in Alzheimer's or Parkinson's disease. In short, precision tools to enable us to predict, track and intervene earlier and more powerfully.

Pharmaceutical innovation—new frontiers of therapy design

We have come a long way since the era of patent medicines. From this era came a fascinating little book I recently came across in an old library. It was called 'Secret Remedies—what they cost and what they contain'—published by the British Medical Association a century ago. Russell's Anti-Corpulent Preparation, available in 12 and a half ounce bottles for the princely sum of six shillings, proved to be simply a solution of citric acid, a common constituent of citrus fruits, coloured with a little iron!

Since those far-off days of medicinal quackery, the worldwide pharmaceutical enterprise has brought us wave after wave of real invention in the form of powerful **chemical drugs**. We have antibiotics for most bacterial infections, ulcer treatments that make stomach surgery for this painful condition a thing of the past, cancer therapies that have turned many cancers into survivable illnesses, and statins and anti-hypertensives that reduce the risk of heart attack and stroke.

Over the last 20 years, designer drugs, specifically shaped to fit known pockets in the proteins involved in disease, have largely replaced those found by trial and error.

HIV has been transformed from a death sentence into a chronic illness, through anti-virals that tackle the virus in several ways. One class of drug blocks the enzyme (the 'protease') that cuts the protein chain coded by the virus gene into its functional components inside the cell it has invaded. Once this protein had been isolated, crystallized and analysed by X-rays, scientists had its precise three-dimensional structure. The design of molecules that could bind and block its 'active site' (the business end of the molecule) could then begin. Picture the docking between a space capsule and the mother ship – in this case the HIV drug and the target.

'Docking' software can now be used to predict how tightly different drugs bind and how resistance to the drug might develop. All of this, like much drug research, now takes place at a computer terminal rather than in the laboratory!

With so many drugs already developed, have we drained the well of possibilities? Far from it. Drug designers, as they work on the thousands of proteins not yet the target of drugs, have at their disposal an unimaginably large number of possible chemical structures involving the atoms carbon, nitrogen and oxygen—the main constituents of drugs. The combinations are estimated at 10^{62} (ten multiplied by itself 62 times!): more than all the atoms in the universe! Perhaps that is why chemists talk of 'exploring chemical space' as they select a drug design as specific for the task as possible.

The binding of the drug to its intended target is only one factor in its effectiveness. It needs to reach its target, by being absorbed via the stomach or through the bloodstream, and not meet a barrier on the way to the cells involved in the disease. It must also stay for long enough at a safe and effective level in the body, broken down at a reasonable rate, so avoiding the opposite fates of either disappearing before it can take effect, or building up to dangerous levels with each successive dose.

No wonder we need to create hundreds of permutations before finding a drug that is safe and effective. Another type of HIV drug, maraviroc, prevents the virus from binding and entering the target cell in the human immune system by blocking a specific (CCR5) receptor. The team at Pfizer working on the drug needed to make and test over 700 variations on the first candidate medicine discovered, before they came up with the best. But the battle against HIV continues: sustained creativity and commitment is needed to find new ways to defeat the virus as it develops resistance to the existing drug arsenal.

Jane's daughter **Caroline** was strong and sporty. She hardly had a day off work, as a practice nurse in the local primary care clinic, but one evening she went early to bed with a high fever. It seemed a scratch on her arm had become infected with a bacterium picked up at the clinic, one that—as shown by genetic and antibiotic resistance tests—would not respond to the normal broad-spectrum antibiotics.

Fortunately for her, and thousands of others, about 12 years earlier a private-public consortium had been set up to fund the development of a new generation of antibiotics that would be kept in reserve specifically for cases of extreme antibiotic resistance. Several pharmaceutical companies had collaborated with the National Institutes of Health in the US and the Wellcome Trust in the UK to produce antibiotics that would not have a normal commercial market and so would not have been developed by the private sector alone.

As soon as the organism infecting Caroline had been matched with its specific antibiotic this was couriered to her doctor and a short course of treatment had her back on her feet in a couple of days. And back on the tennis court shortly after.

New medicines can also come from broadening or redirecting existing drugs. PARP inhibitors, first developed for a specific type of cancer (caused by the BRCA1 and 2 mutations which predispose some women to breast cancer), turn out to accelerate the death of a wide variety of cancer cells by interfering with their DNA repair mechanisms. So, serendipity is still a potent force in drug discovery.

A whole new approach to medicines development has opened up in the last 20 to 30 years. **Biological agents**, either identical or similar to the body's own proteins, have transformed several areas of medicine. A few were already available from natural sources, like insulin from pigs, or human growth hormone from the pituitary glands of human cadavers. But when scientists discovered 'recombinant DNA' technology, incorporating the right human genes into fast growing cells like bacteria, they found they could produce synthetic 'human' proteins identical or similar to the body's own, in unlimited quantities.

Among the most powerful have been **monoclonal antibodies**. They direct the action of specific human antibodies against the rogue cells and proteins involved in disease. For example, in the debilitating disease of rheumatoid arthritis, tissues over-react to a growth factor called TNF. Antibodies against this protein slow the progress of this form of arthritis quite dramatically, and restore a near-normal life to patients suffering severe pain and loss of mobility.

Monoclonals themselves have now entered the 'designer' era. Wide varieties of human-compatible ('humanized') antibodies are generated and screened to get the best fit to the target, before any are made at commercial scale. Biological drugs are more expensive than chemical drugs as they must be produced by fermentation in micro-organisms.

Long-established biological agents are, of course, **vaccines**. The practice of injecting mild or deactivated forms of a virus into patients to prepare them to combat the real thing goes back to Edward Jenner and his work on smallpox in 1796. But moving from identifying the pathogen to creating an effective vaccine has been a long and uncertain affair. It took 45 years between the identification of the polio virus in 1909 and the first vaccine in 1954; now the disease has been essentially eradicated in the developed world. Three disease-causing viruses were discovered in the 1970s (rotavirus, hepatitis A, and HPV, the virus that causes cervical cancer) but it still took between 22 and 33 years to create the right vaccines for these infections. Twenty-five years after the identification of the HIV virus we still await a vaccine, although there are about 20 possibilities under study.

However, once we have developed an effective vaccine to a class of viruses, we can now respond very rapidly to a new strain emerging. It took only four months to develop the first vaccine to the 2009 strain of H1N1 influenza. The steps for this turbocharged vaccine development are shown in Figure 1.1.

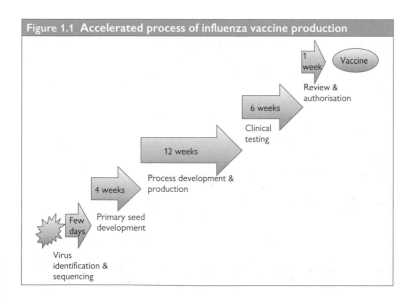

Figure 1.1 Accelerated process of influenza vaccine production

1 week → Vaccine

Review & authorisation

6 weeks

Clinical testing

12 weeks

Process development & production

4 weeks

Primary seed development

Few days

Virus identification & sequencing

A major advance in vaccine development has been the design of adjuvants—large molecules coupled to the vaccine 'antigens' to multiply the body's response. In the critical challenge of quickly creating enough influenza vaccine from a new strain, multiplying the effect of limited quantities of antigen can make all the difference between being able to quickly vaccinate the whole population and protecting just a small proportion.

The most exciting recent addition to the vaccine armoury is the concept of the DNA vaccine—providing the DNA ingredients to boost the body's own resistance to disease. In multiple sclerosis, T-cells from the immune system attack the outer protective layer of nerve cells—the so-called myelin sheath – which helps the nerves conduct their electrical messages. One of the targets for this misguided T-cell attack is a protein called MBP (Myelin Basic Protein). A vaccine containing the gene for MBP production is now in trials and showing some effect in reducing brain lesions in MS patients.

Our growing knowledge of gene function has opened up the possibility of 'silencing' them, using **small interfering RNA molecules** (siRNAs). These very precise inhibitors stop the translation of their target genes into proteins by 'interfering' with the genetic message en route to the cell's protein production factories. They are already useful tools to explore what specific genes do, and commercial companies are now offering 'gene silencers' for most of the genes that code for protein production.

The future hope is that siRNA drugs will be able to specifically target disease-associated genes as precisely as monoclonal antibodies knock out disease-associated proteins. The challenge will not be making the siRNA, it will be in delivering it to the target cell, without the body's enzymes breaking it down before it gets there. One approach is to bind the active agent to a nanoparticle containing a cell-specific molecule on its outer surface.

Susannah's father–in-law **Don** had his annual physical exam with the service specified by his personal health plan. He always made time in his schedule for this, even though it took the best part of a day. Not only did his wife Abigail insist on it, the plan credited him with premium points if he had the check within 15 months of his last one. He felt well, and there was nothing untoward on the day, so he was surprised and concerned when his primary care doctor called a few days later. He told him that the blood tests indicated prostate cancer at an early stage, but of a kind that should not be left to develop further.

Scans indicated the tumour was small, so Don was placed on a new 'siRNA' drug that had successfully eliminated prostate cancers of just this genetic profile. The drug silenced a gene that was essential for cell division and hence the growth of the tumour. Along with a medicine that boosted the body's own rejection of the cancerous cells, the drug ensured that, when Don was re-scanned just three months later, no sign of either the tumour or any circulating cancer cells could be found.

The early prospects for siRNA therapy are good when the delivery challenge is not too great. For example lung disease can be treated with inhaled agent without the complications of protecting and targeting an injected drug. One of the pioneer companies in this area has already safety-tested an siRNA agent to protect lung transplant patients against the respiratory virus RSV.

Where will the therapeutic frontiers be in the coming years? We can already see some way into this future: since pharmaceuticals take a decade or more to move from test-tube to patient, the 10-year future is clearer than in most other areas of innovation, where the product cycles are much shorter. This snapshot of the future is called the 'pharmaceutical pipeline'. So, 10 years ahead we know to expect ever more targeted and better tolerated cancer medicines, new drugs to slow and even reverse arthritis and other immune disorders, and antibiotics to deal with the growing number of resistant strains of bacteria, like MRSA and C difficile.

If we look 20 years ahead, beyond today's pipeline, where can we expect advances? We recently pooled the thinking of several pharmaceutical companies on this question, for a dialogue with the UK government. The answers were interesting. The experts foresaw appetite suppressors, drugs to boost immune response to infection and new approaches to Alzheimer's disease. We will also see, I'm sure, therapies based on siRNA gene silencing in clinical trials.

A controversial frontier will be the creation of 'nootropic' drugs to enhance normal brain function. Will we see such agents to turn man into superman—with greater powers of concentration, speed of thinking and depth of memory? We already have agents that reverse the damage of disease on these functions, and widespread use by the healthy of caffeine, nicotine, and amphetamines and other 'brain steroids', as they are called in online magazines. One in five scientists and researchers were recently reported to be using brain-enhancing substances!

So it is entirely possible that in 20 years we may see regulatory acceptance of the use of nootropic drugs to make normal brain function super-normal, or—perhaps more acceptably—to retain normal mental function in the aging brain.

Drugs, both chemical and biological, and vaccines will play a major role in the therapeutic drama over the next 20 years. But they will be joined by a completely new strand of innovation, in which we coax our own genes and cells to become powerful therapeutic agents.

Regenerative medicine—genes and cells to the rescue

The London Underground has a famous 'Mind the Gap' warning. There should be a similar warning for bioscience investors and commentators: there is always a gap of about 20 years between the initial flurry of publicity for a new

15

therapeutic technology and its real impact on routine medicine. It has applied to the different waves of pharmaceutical innovation we have just explored— for example, antibodies, discovered in the 60s and 70s, initially proposed as 'magic bullet' pharmaceuticals in the 80s, did not come into broad use until the 90s and beyond.

The same is likely to be true for both gene and stem cell therapy. Selecting agents with the right therapeutic properties, reducing side-effects, delivering them to the site of action and then testing them rigorously for safety and efficacy will be major challenges.

Gene therapy was off the starting blocks in the early 90s, but hit troubling technical problems and saw a few patient deaths in its earliest trials. So no gene therapy is yet formally approved by the US medicines regulator, the FDA.

In principle, the concept is simple. If a patient lacks a gene, or the right form of a gene, then why not insert it directly into the cells that need it, or insert a regulator gene to switch the patient's own genes on or off in the 'right' way?

As we discover the functions of more and more genes, applications of this approach seem endless, from metabolic deficiencies, through cancer to HIV. The main challenge is getting the gene inserted in the patient's cells, a step that requires the use of a 'vector' (typically a benign virus) to carry the gene. There is a high risk of the body rejecting the combination. More worrying is the risk that interfering with the patient's genome could trigger other diseases of genetic origin, like leukemia.

Therefore, for gene therapy, we are still in the 'gap' – but perhaps not for much longer. In early 2008, the first gene therapy trials for a type of inherited blindness were successful in London's Moorfields Eye Hospital. In this disease (Leber's Congenital Amaurosis), the patient inherits an abnormal form of the gene called RPE65. The experimental treatment inserted the correct version of the gene into the patient's retina and, in the case of one teenage patient, achieved a real improvement in night vision, with no obvious side effects.

Gene therapy also looks promising as a way of converting, or 'reprogramming' one type of cell into another. Inserting the right transcription genes into one type of cell in the pancreas, the exocrine cells, can convert them into the precious beta cells that are needed to manufacture insulin to combat diabetes. At least they do in mice!

Similar encouragement is being seen in trials on blood cancers, where targeting the genes is simpler than for solid tumours. Liposomes (small lipid envelopes) deliver genes into cell nuclei, by-passing the troublesome use of viruses as vectors. In this 'medical nanotechnology' a single gene is wrapped in a lipid envelope just 25 nanometres in size.

Cell therapy takes the replacing/renewing approach one step further – inserting whole human cells to replace those that have been lost or become dysfunctional, as a result of disease, injury or ageing. This approach has been used successfully, employing a patient's own cells, for some time—in bone marrow transplants for cancer patients. These cells, vital to sustain the immune system, that would otherwise be killed by chemotherapy, are withdrawn before drug treatment begins, and then re-injected once it is complete.

However, the breakthrough in this area in recent years has been the controversial **stem cell technology**. Initially derived from unwanted human embryonic tissue, stem cells can develop ('differentiate') into a wide variety of tissue cells. So, in principle, new pancreatic, nerve, heart or brain cells could be inserted to restore insulin manufacture, nerve connections, heart muscle or proper motor control.

The ethics of embryonic stem cell (ESC) research have received a great deal of attention. The debate was focused by the Bush Administration's decision to ban federally funded ESC research that used cell lines other than those already existing when the law was passed. Many others around the world (and indeed other research funders in the USA) did not have the same concerns. However, the ethical issues would largely disappear if 'pluripotent' stem cells (derived from adult tissue) turn out to be as effective.

Stem cell therapy possibilities read like medical science fiction – new organs, new nerve connections, even restored brain function. Recently a functioning arterial blood vessel was grown from a section of skin! In some cases, a patient's own stem cells are being used to coat a tissue graft from a donor, so as to increase the likelihood that the graft will be successful. To illustrate these future possibilities, a single weekly edition of Cell Therapy News (November 16, 2009) reported: the restoration of limb function after spinal cord injuries, reprogramming the specialized immune cells called B-cells into macrophages to attack infection, the restoration of memory or learning deficits after radiation therapy for brain tumours, a possible treatment for Duchenne Muscular Dystrophy and Parkinson's disease. Although most of these announcements are for animal studies, the issue also reported human Phase 2 clinical trials for the use of cardiac repair cells to treat severe chronic heart failure.

Susannah's mother-in-law, **Abigail**, is a robust and matronal figure. But when she began to become unaccountably breathless the specialist diagnosed a severe constriction in her left lung as a result of fibrosis (scar tissue building up from a previous infection) in the airway. While the lung itself was quite healthy it was essentially useless.

The first step was to find a matched donor for that part of the lung. Then cells that had been removed from Abigail's own skin and converted into stem cells were used to coat the implant before it was inserted in her lung. The result was a much more reliable replacement and a complete restoration of her lung function within weeks. Like glue on a repair, the cells cemented the new part lastingly into place.

Whatever the source of the cells, 'regenerative medicine' using stem cells will surely bring its own crop of practical problems. Techniques to coax the cell lines to mimic the cells in a particular organ are far from being mastered, except in a few cases. And the scale-up and manufacturing challenges will be substantial: growing human cells outside the body, keeping them genetically stable and in good condition for therapy are complicated steps that will not be a matter of routine for some time.

Before that arrives, we will see stem cells helping in the development of other treatments. I chair a UK-based company Stem Cells for Safer Medicines (SC4SM), developing stem cells as a source of liver and heart cells. The goal is to test new drugs on these cell lines to mimic their behaviour in the two organs most often responsible for the unwanted side-effects of medicines. The result should be fewer potential drugs dropping out because of liver or heart toxicity.

In the USA, cells from individuals with 10 different genetic diseases have been 'reprogrammed' with viruses to produce stem cells. Such cell lines will enable both closer study of the molecular basis of disease and also the testing of therapies on near-human tissue.

So much for the science. The ultimate challenge for both gene and cell therapy will probably be economic. Chemical drugs, once developed, are relatively cheap to make and administer—their prices can be high to recover high R&D costs during the life of the drug patent, but administering the pill or injection does not carry a high cost. However, in gene and cell therapy, the individual treatment doses and patient procedures are likely to be complex and cost tens of thousands of dollars per patient, at least for some time. Economics, rather than technology, may prove the greatest barrier to their routine use.

Images and imaging—seeing ourselves as never before

A range of remarkable imaging techniques can now bring us pictures of how the human body functions, in health and disease—with exquisite insight, detail and often beauty. The techniques may have impenetrable names—computerized tomography (CT), magnetic resonance imaging (MRI), and positron emission tomography (PET)—but they are able to penetrate the body and reveal what we have never seen before.

The oldest technology, X-rays, developed into **CT (computerized tomography) scanning**. This images parts and thin slices of the body and so builds up a three-dimensional picture of an organ and its internal structure. A spiral CT scan of the heart identifies the level of calcium buildup in the coronary arteries, a sign of plaque formation prior to a potential heart attack. CT scans can spot abnormalities, such as tumours, in most internal organs.

Magnetic resonance imaging (MRI) has developed dramatically from the time of my own PhD research into biological magnetic resonance. MRI provides high resolution images of the softer tissues, such as the brain or nervous system, not well visualized by CT scans. It therefore gives a precise spatial picture of a problem that could not be gained in any other way.

As well as joint and spine injury, this technology is also very good for diagnosis of tumours in the softer tissues. The images of the brain are quite beautiful, and give the surgeon an extremely precise guide, vitally important for neurosurgery.

If the position of a brain tumour is known, but it is difficult or impossible to remove by surgery, there is a new option—the **gamma knife**. Here the patient wears a special helmet that enables gamma rays from 201 different radioactive sources to be directed to the same point in the brain. This kills the tumour or removes an aneurism while keeping the rest of the brain relatively spared from radiation. Without the accurate MRI imaging, of course, this therapy would be impossible.

'Functional MRI' uses pulses of radiofrequency to track changes in the image over time. It reveals dynamic changes in the tissues – for example blood flow in the brain or the changes in heart muscle biochemistry during exercise. Blood flow studies are showing how, even in young brains, the use of drugs, or even too much caffeine, can slow or cut off the blood supply to parts of the brain, with disastrous long term consequences.

MRI on normal brains, showing which areas 'light up' when we are frightened or aroused, enables us to link our behaviour and our moods with our brain chemistry. Older people are told to keep their brains working—MRI can show the impact of reading, writing and surfing (the web, of course!) on the areas of the brain that are kept alert.

PET scanning—positron emission tomography—is the newest of the 'big three' imaging technologies. Tracer substances containing a short-lived radioisotope are injected into the body, and the concentration of the tracer is tracked by the gamma rays it emits. If the tracer is a form of glucose, PET scanning reveals the level of metabolism in an organ (showing how active it is). If the tracer is a labelled medicine, PET can track how the drug distributes itself around the body. PET is often combined with CT scanning to improve the reconstruction of the image and identification of disease.

All of these techniques are becoming steadily better in terms of their resolution (how fine the image is), their convenience and their cost. Convenience for the patient is not just a matter of closeness to home, but also the comfort of the procedure. Early MRI scanners were both noisy and claustrophobic: now 'open' MRI scanners can avoid the claustrophobia, and 'peripheral' machines can scan knees and ankles while the patient sits in a chair and reads a newspaper! We even have 'intra-operative' MRI imaging during surgery itself, allowing surgeons to check they have removed all of a brain tumour before closing up the patient's skull!

Images are often enhanced by substances that are injected to improve the contrast and definition of the image. Magnetic nanoparticles are being used to track the spread of cancer and to distinguish affected lymph nodes from those that remain normal. This provides the surgeon with a colour-coded map showing the healthy versus cancerous tissue, while surgery is still underway.

What will we see in the next 20 years as a result of these steady improvements in imaging? We can envisage a time when annual MRI scans can be used to detect changes from one year to the next that might be the first warning signs of disease. Or, for cancer sufferers in remission, regular PET scans will spot the smallest recurrence anywhere in the body. As the volume of such tests goes up, the costs will come down to levels that will make them an affordable part of the annual physical examination.

Novel combinations of scans with electrical sensors will offer new insights, especially in the brain. Recent research combines MRI images of the brain with EEG electrical signals. This combination will be better at locating the source of epileptic disturbances than either technique alone, so more precise treatment can be planned.

Jane had a bad scare just a couple of years ago, when her father **Peter** started to suffer mysterious headaches, despite his annual MRI scan showing no obvious abnormality. He then began to have odd hallucinations and attacks of dizziness. After a day at the nearest advanced imaging centre they had done linked EEG-MRI scanning and an arteriogram and spotted an arteriovenous malformation (AVM) or nidus—a fragile tangle of blood vessels that was ready to cause a major haemorrhage.

The same day they strapped on a 'gamma knife' helmet and were ready to direct a precision beam of radiation to seal off the vessels and prevent a catastrophic stroke. But because of the delicate location of the lesion, the team video-linked in a specialist at the gamma knife centre in Charlottesville, Virginia, who had done or directed literally hundreds of these procedures, to check the settings and number of radiation 'shots' against his experience, and against the accumulated database of successful outcomes on all previous procedures in that part of the brain.

Finally, we will see new ways of using the images in the process of surgery, projecting the results of the internal scan on to the body of a patient undergoing surgery, so that the surgeon can insert catheters or deliver therapy to the precise spot in three dimensions indicated by the scan.

More new scanning technologies will emerge over the next 20 years. For example, Raman spectroscopy stands today where PET stood 20 years ago. Raman researchers, who measure the scattering of laser light from biological samples, claim that it will have a much finer ultimate resolution and be able to visualize many different types of molecules. The first experiments have linked tumour-hunting antibodies to tiny (nano-) particles of gold and uses laser light to highlight where the particles migrate. Visualizing microscopic tumours will be a tremendous help to the surgeon aiming to remove all abnormal tissue.

All of these imaging technologies require very expensive capital equipment—from a few hundred thousand pounds or dollars to many millions. PET scanning, in particular, requires an on-site cyclotron to produce radioisotopes, and ultra-fast chemical synthesis to turn them in minutes into the molecule that is to be injected. So PET is still typically found only in major medical centres, while CT and MRI scanners are now routinely seen in community-based clinics, at least in the USA.

Personalized Medicine—every treatment made to measure

We are all unique individuals—a unique combination of height, hair and eye colour, body shape and skills, to name but a few of our more obvious personal characteristics. So it should be no surprise that we each suffer disease in different forms and respond differently to treatments.

Oliver Sachs, the distinguished physician and author of many entertaining books on psychiatry, once said: 'Don't just ask what disease this patient has, ask what patient the disease has!' He might have added: 'Don't just ask if this therapy is right for the disease, ask if it is right for this patient.'

Until recently we lacked the tools to turn that insight about our uniqueness into better medicine, more precisely tuned to individual need. Now a wide range of personalizing tools are beginning to be forged: our personal gene sequence holds the key to our predisposition to develop a given disease, and molecular markers in our blood provide pointers to our likely response to the drugs developed to treat it.

The complete sequence of a human genome is still an expensive and laborious business. The sequencing of the first genomes to be completed—those of Craig Venter (founder of the company Celera) and James Watson (discoverer of the double helix of DNA) took 10 years and billions of dollars. In the year 2000 the full sequence was published for the first time, to much fanfare.

By 2008 a commercial company called Knome ('Know-me') was offering individual customers their own sequence for a mere $250,000! Within a year the price had dropped to a trifling $99,500. However, for this a customer receives not only the sequence but a counseling service that explains the significance of all the main variations of the individual's genome from the 'standard' version.

Cheaper options are available: a company called 23andMe offers sequencing at 500,000 points on a customer's genome, reporting on 20 to 30 genes – for $1,000 per person. The tests focus on mitochondrial (i.e. maternal) DNA and Y-chromosome (i.e. paternal) DNA, highlighting which characteristics come from which parent.

New ways of tagging specific parts of the genome, plus new ways to automate the sequencing around them, and rapid computerized information processing will soon bring us the $1,000 genome. We will be able to know the

30 billion letters in each child's genome soon after birth. What are the implications? What will we do with the information?

We are all familiar to some extent with genetic diseases. Haemophilia blighted all the male descendants of Queen Victoria. Huntingdon's disease afflicts half the offspring of couples one of whom has the abnormal HD gene. These diseases result from a single genetic error on one particular gene. However, most diseases are polygenic—many genes interact with each other and with the environment in and out of the body to determine whether a disease appears. So in most cases what the genetic information will tell us is the rough probability that an individual will contract the disease.

But should we use the tools to determine this probability? Or, a better question: at what stages in life, and for what conditions, does it make sense? The answer is simple—whenever the risk of conducting the test is in proportion to the health risk involved in the disease and something concrete can be done with the result—in other words eliminate, reduce or postpone the disease's impact, through preventative medicine.

One example—doctors in Australia have developed a test for predisposition to a form of meningitis, which indicates whether someone is likely to develop the disease, and therefore should be vaccinated. Of course, genetic information about predisposition can be a mixed blessing, if a disease is still incurable, or a breach of confidentiality puts the data in the wrong hands. But in most cases it will enable the individual to lead a longer and healthier life.

We need to dispel one myth—that our genome spells a precise destiny for each one of us. If it did, of course, there would be no point in making the right lifestyle choices. The fact is that how we live our lives can have a profound influence on how the genes express themselves—the difference between the so-called genotype (what we could become) and our phenotype (what we actually become, as a result of everything we ask our bodies to do and the environment they are exposed to).

To make the most of our new-found ability to link genetic make-up with disease we will need access to large-scale 'tissue banks' such as the one now being assembled in the UK—the BioBank. It has already stored blood from nearly 400,000 volunteers, in the world's largest storage facility of its kind, so that studies can be done to establish the links to guide future research and therapy.

As a result of efforts like this worldwide, our awareness of our genes, and their implications for who we are, is mounting by the day. This results in a stream of news items—many of questionable scientific value. In addition to genes for anger, sexual orientation, and so on, a recent article described how our reaction to horror films is controlled by the 'COMT' gene. Two copies of the Met158 version of the gene (the 'anxiety mutation') apparently makes the individual easily horrified and thus unable (perhaps fortunately for them) to watch the worst horror movies!

Rather more useful are the studies to highlight when a patient's genetic makeup puts them at risk of a serious side effect from drug treatment. An international Serious Adverse Events Consortium (SAEC) has been set up to probe just such effects. The SAEC, established in October 2007, is a non-profit entity comprising large pharmaceutical companies, research organizations such as the Wellcome Trust, and regulatory bodies like the FDA. Work funded by the SAEC recently discovered that a specific genotype (HLA-B5701) makes patients a hundred times more vulnerable to liver damage when taking the common antibiotic flucloxacillin.

Despite these rapid advances, talk of 'personalized' medicine is a bit over-ambitious. The dream of an individual drug at an individual dose in an individual regimen is unaffordable and usually unnecessary. Most of the time we are talking about better targeted therapy, which some call 'stratified medicine'. A test or a battery of tests is used to decide whether someone is in a subgroup of the population that will best respond to drug A, or should get drug B instead.

There is debate about what kinds of routine tests will prove most useful. '**Pharmacogenetic**' tests home in on sections of the genome characteristic of the disease or the drug response, and query it using gene probes. One of the common HIV medicines, abacavir, triggers sometimes fatal hypersensitivity in a small minority (8%) of patients, but almost all of the problem can be predicted and avoided by testing for a particular form of the B5701 gene in patients' white blood cells.

'**Proteomic**' tests focus on proteins that provide a molecular fingerprint for a sub-type of a disease. We now know that sepsis, the condition that kills many patients in intensive care, varies widely in the pattern of molecular events taking place in the patient's bloodstream. Proteomic tests can tell us which patients are in greatest danger and which of these will respond to the only drug treatment currently available, Xigris.

'**Metabolomic**' tests assess the levels of circulating metabolites that are associated with variations of a disease. This is the simplest of the molecular signatures at our disposal, and the basis of most 'blood tests': a familiar example is the measurement of glucose to diagnose diabetes and determine if a diabetic needs an injection of insulin. More complex signatures, involving several markers, are likely to be needed for true targeted therapy. But they may be much less expensive than genetic or proteomic alternatives costing hundreds of pounds or dollars each.

Personalizing tests will guide medical treatment, but may also guide the design of personalized nutrition. '**Nutrigenomics**' creates and promotes foods or combinations of foods to match the health risks of individuals. If such foods come with specific health claims, they will need to be backed up by clinical studies. Such trials, always run by pharmaceutical innovators, are foreign to food manufacturers, but we may well see them in the years to come.

In its infancy, personalized medicine will probably be of greatest value in combating cancer – a personalized disease, because it is fundamentally a disorder of the patient's own genome. Genes are switched on (or off) that create a line of cells within the body with different, and often disastrous, growth characteristics. The International Cancer Genome Consortium is a $600 million project to identify all the mutations that drive the 50 most common forms of cancer.

Once the genetic fingerprint of a patient's tumour has been determined from a biopsy, personalized treatment in the form of specific drug cocktails, can be designed. We can also use protein markers (like Her-2-neu) to distinguish whether a protein-specific drug (in this case Herceptin) will inhibit growth. Cancer treatment progress can also be tracked by blood tests for the specific genetic rearrangements in circulating cancer cells, thanks to technology developed at Johns Hopkins University.

Genetic analysis of tumour tissues has brought another valuable insight into the relationship between various different cancers. In the past we have described cancers in terms of the organ in which they begin—breast, colon, lung, prostate, etc. But genetic analysis reveals that the underlying genetic errors in some colon cancers have more in common with some prostate cancers than other tumours of the colon. This opens up the exciting possibility that some of the newest generation of targeted drugs for cancer A will also work in some patients with cancer B, because of the disease mechanisms and drug targets they have in common.

Jane's mother, **Grace**, was one of the first of her generation to insist on starting screening for colon cancer when in her 50s. There were several possibilities—a full colonoscopy, a sigmoidoscopy to probe only the 'descending' part of the colon, genetic tests on the faeces, and blood tests to spot circulating proteins associated with cancer. They all had different sensitivity (the assurance that a cancer is not missed) and specificity (the risk of 'false positives' – positive results that cause worry and further investigation but turn out to be misleading). Since she had no symptoms and disliked the idea of the preparation for a colonoscopy, she chose a stool test, and it showed a positive.

This meant that a full colonoscopy was now unavoidable, and it showed an early stage tumour. Caught quite early, the best course was simply to have surgery, and then do a full genetic profiling of the tumour tissue. This was a full sequencing of those parts of the tumour genes that showed what type of genetic errors had occurred and gave a clear prognosis.

The genetic test revealed that this was an aggressive type, and that any remaining cells that might be in the body had a high chance of creating a dangerous metastatic cancer. Grace was referred to a genetic oncologist who used the profile to create the exact cocktail of drugs that would be most effective in preventing further cancer growth.

Having had her op fifteen years ago and completing the oral drug therapy the following year, Grace had been cancer-free ever since.

Beyond the area of cancer, DNA tests (for example GeneSightRx tests from AssureRx) are now on offer to distinguish patients most likely to respond to anti-depressants. Imaging can also be used to distinguish patients likely to respond: severely depressed patients usually have a lower level of function in a specific part of the brain called the anterior cingulate cortex. MRI studies have demonstrated a link between the activity in this part of the brain and response to the most common anti-depressants, the Selective Serotonin Reuptake Inhibitors (SSRIs).

Within 20 years we can expect most conditions to have diagnostic tests to distinguish different types of disease and predict patient response, to guide treatment decisions. But the ultimate destination will be a personalised health plan for each one of us, based on knowledge of the most likely disease risks, given our genes, and the changes of diet, exercise and medication that will maximize our chances of avoiding them. And, if disease develops, tests will reveal the sub-group to which we belong, which therapy is best, and the treatment regimen to suit our age, weight, metabolism and lifestyle.

Such personalized care plans will finally put us in the 'driving seat', that is if we wish to take the wheel of our own health journey. Not everyone will, of course, but patient engagement is that much more likely if we know the therapy has been tailor-made for us, rather than just 'off the peg'.

However, personal predictive plans will not come cheap. Full gene sequences, protein profiles of disease progress and tests to predict drug response will all be expensive upfront investments to guide more precise treatment.

Healthcare information—from data to knowledge

Healthcare has long been bedeviled by information gaps, errors, and duplication. We need only to think of the number of times we have been asked for the same information (date of birth, allergies, chronic conditions, family history) as we journey through the healthcare system. And of the tragic consequences of many of the all-too-frequent errors in choice of medication or of dose.

The fact we are being asked the same questions over and over again, and that errors are often still made, is a sure sign there is no real information 'system' at all. A US Health Secretary recently declared that the availability of a shareable electronic medical record is the first sign he will take that the fragmented US non-system is actually being woven into a real healthcare system.

I once worked for IBM, for the man credited with bringing the company back from the brink of being broken up into various parts. Chairman Lou Gerstner realised that, in the old IBM adage, 'it's how we pull it together that sets us apart.' I headed IBM's healthcare sector, which seemed to me to have a special place on the chairman's radar screen. His own experience and that of his family, drove home to him how desperately fragmented is our healthcare information. 'It's how it's *not* pulled together that sets it apart', in fact.

Why, we ask, do we need to fill in the same medical details, on a different form, on a different clipboard, whenever we visit a doctor for the first time? Why do doctors so often repeat blood tests, or x-rays, because past results are unavailable? Why does the information system in the general practitioner's office not talk to the one in the local hospital?

The answers are actually quite simple. Past investments in information systems have been made to collect information for financial reimbursement purposes, or to compile public health statistics, or to ease the working life of a particular part of the hospital, like pathology or radiology. Each purpose-built system captured a different aspect of the patient journey: getting an overall picture of a patient's care was not a high priority.

As healthcare IT has spread its wings, it has begun to tackle this problem—with the electronic medical record (EMR). The EMR is designed to pull together the disparate fragments of the patient's diagnosis and treatment, slowly replacing the old manila folders—with their loose sheets of scribbled notes.

There are, however, some fundamental problems with achieving the 'Holy Grail' of integrated healthcare information at the doctor's fingertips. Most important, from the technical standpoint, is the sheer diversity of types and sources of data they need to contain: X-ray images, yes/no allergy information, numerical test results, typed referral letters, prescriptions for drugs, handwritten or dictated physical exam notes, and on and on. Any or none of these may be relevant to a particular consultation with a doctor.

A second major issue is the challenge of inserting computer-based tools into the doctor-patient conversation. Few doctors can refer to them and update them with ease with the patient in front of them, without it distracting them or slowing them down. And for doctors, time-efficiency is all important. A third barrier is ambiguous information: different descriptions for diseases or drugs, or uncertainty about patient identification.

Over the next 20 years, both technology and market forces will solve these problems. Web-based software tools will overcome the compatibility barriers to moving information around the system. And major health systems will see that improving their performance, both clinically and financially, will depend crucially on integrated information.

Standards will emerge to enable EMR systems to share information with each other, and for the critical parts of the record of each patient to be loaded on a smart card chip. These cards will then be, just as bank cards have been for years, a passport for the patient as she accesses every part of the system. It will also store personal health data like exercise regimens and nutrition programmes.

A lifelong medical record, accessible on appropriate authority, to anyone in any location, will move from a 'Holy Grail' to a daily reality.

We will also see the design of other electronic tools that doctors find a real help, not a hindrance. Denmark's national Patient Health Portal already enables communication and services to flow between health professionals and citizens, including booking of appointments with GPs, conducting e-mail consultations and renewing prescriptions. A new French system, 'Diabcarnet', monitors diabetics via the first large-scale electronic logbook for a disease, enabling patients to partner with their physicians to manage their disease.

Treatment guidelines are available for complex, multi-choice conditions such as cancer. In the US, the National Comprehensive Cancer Center Network guidelines cover many huge sheets of paper, giving the options and best choices at multiple points in the course of the disease. But few doctors want to leaf through these with an anxious patient in their office. A company that I once led delivered such guidelines for cancer direct to the desktop of oncologists: it now steers care in no less than 417 sites around the USA. Over the next 20 years such 'decision support systems' will become standard in all major clinical areas.

'NHS Evidence' is now setting out to create a decision support resource for the UK across all common conditions. The goal is to have the information available at the point of decision-making (on an 'information pull' basis), since it is well known that doctors cannot absorb all they might need from 'information push' media like medical journals. Such comprehensive evidence-based information will not be cheap to produce: about £33 million a year has been allocated to build it over the next few years.

Information systems will also change where and how healthcare is provided. For example patients with a chronic condition, or recently discharged from hospital, can be remotely monitored in their own homes, saving costs and travel stress. Mobile phones can be used to transmit data to a central monitoring point, a technology already available to diabetics for blood glucose tests.

Electronic pill boxes will track whether patients are taking their medication correctly, alerting patient and doctor of missed medications. Such systems will be a tremendous boon for the elderly who easily become confused by multiple medications.

What information revolutions will be built on these foundations in the next 20 years? Let us take a look around the information-enabled health system of 2030.

The first thing we notice is the lack of repetition of the basic information we are so often asked for—past medical and family history, drug allergies, and so on. All of these will be at the doctors', nurses', and receptionists' fingertips, whenever we enter the system, as soon as we give our unique identification number (or provide our healthcare smart card) to verify who we are.

As we look around the doctor's surgery, or outpatient clinic, we will see expert systems to guide the selection of treatment. Drug choices, including contra-indications, costs, and dosage forms will pop up once a diagnosis is made, along with any relevant formularies or other guidelines. Treatment pathways will be suggested, but in a way that the doctor can customize for the individual patient, after she has run the available personalizing tests for the disease.

And once the right pathway is chosen, the system will print out, or send to the patient's e-mail, a patient-friendly description of the disease and the treatment, including answers to all the questions that always occur to us *after* we have left the doctor's surgery. If a referral is being made to a specialist, his or her selection will be based on outcomes and experience of the condition, distance from the patient's home, and the availability of an early appointment. If surgery is needed, both patient and referring doctor will consult the outcomes achieved at that hospital and by that surgeon in comparable cases.

More fundamentally, the information infrastructure we will build will enable the healthcare system to become a 'learning organization'. It will record each patient's characteristics, the care received and the outcome achieved. It will compare treatment and results with the pathways followed by other similar patients, and use this information to decide the best. Commissioning for the care for the next group of patients can then take all this into account—while encouraging innovation where the doctor knows best practice but thinks she can improve upon it. In this case, the system will again assess the outcome, compare it with past best practice and update for the future.

In short we will have a learning system, constantly collecting and sharing information on what works best. From collection of data, to analysis of information, to clinical knowledge. Moving from 'islands of information' in doctors' heads or local IT systems, to a national or international knowledge network.

Future generations of patients will also expect health information at their own fingertips. The Web is already a major source of health information (the Web's second most common use, it is said). However, organizing and accessing it is a challenge, as any simple search for a drug or a disease will show. Inputting 'diabetes' into Google yields 74 million entries, narrowed to a mere 20 million if you specify Type II. If you are a Type II diabetic and want advice on diet there are only 3.8 million sites to review; to find out the effect of foods on your blood sugar you have less than half a million to scan!

As we narrow down to more specific questions, we find many shortlisted responses are from private sites or even health cranks of one kind or another. Enter a request for side effects of a common pharmaceutical for bipolar disorder: the sixth listed of a total of 350,000 sites links you to a class action attorney, just in case you need to sue a doctor or company! We will need trusted sources of well-accredited information.

Information must be personalized to be really useful. The personal portable medical record will become the answer for the coming 'constantly wired' generations. As well as reminding the user to take medicines, or follow an exercise regime, it could accumulate data either automatically (for example, heart rate and rhythm) or by user input (number of calories, or exercise taken). Rapid feedback, both positive and negative, may change our behaviour in a way that our occasional 'must do better' resolutions seem unable to do.

Jane's mother-in-law **Rose** loved to travel. And sometimes to countries that may not be, shall we say, at the top of the advanced medicine experience curve. Her latest exploit was a visit with a friend to a village of the Karin people in the far north of Thailand. She had taken the right anti-malarial for the region, and was enjoying the basic but very warm welcome of the people. Though she usually did not drink, the local brew was very welcome in the heat.

It was while she was there that she started to experience diarrhoea and took a broad spectrum antibiotic she had picked up in Bangkok in case of just such an event. But she went from bad to worse. First she had a bad rash on her face and chest and then became very feverish.

She used her mobile phone to call her physician in Chicago, but of course it was the middle of the night there. However, the answering service, on hearing the symptoms, suggested she text the names of the drugs she was taking to the drug-drug interaction checker, that was automatically linked to the results of her drug metabolism profile. This told the doctor—or in this case the automated system—that she was deficient in one of the common pathways for drug metabolism, the 2D6 cytochrome p450 pathway, and that the combination of drugs she was taking, particularly after alcohol, was overloading her system. It also carried the reminder that she was taking an anti-depressant that made matters worse.

She received a text in a matter of minutes, telling her which medication to stop and what to do if the symptoms did not improve. She survived the ordeal and made a mental note for the future to discuss what she might need to take before leaving home.

Better healthcare information is much more than a luxury—information gaps can kill. I once served on the board of directors of a medical informatics company. The doctor-founder of the company tells the story of when he was a young doctor on call at a major hospital. One night he found that a patient was about to be given a drug to which he was dangerously allergic, and stopped the administration of the drug just in time. He ordered that a large sign be put above the bed prohibiting the drug.

But, like many such paper notices, it went missing. The next time he was called to the patient's bedside, it was to certify his death—from administration of the very same drug. That moment he determined to make better online medical information the goal of his career.

Smart devices—going where no man has gone before

A mainstay of science fiction books and films has long been bionic implants replacing, enhancing or controlling the body's own function. In the real world, artificial joints and heart pacemakers started the field. Soon stents arrived to hold open arteries, and implantable defibrillators to startle the heart back into action when it falters. Pain blocking devices have proven their worth when nervous systems are damaged by injury. And now there is talk of implantable devices that detect the first electrical signs of an epileptic fit and prevent the seizure before it happens.

Many devices are developed by ingenious surgeons and other interventionists. As an advisor to the Boston Childrens' Hospital I saw new ideas come thick and fast, from a simple device to measure skull shape accurately, to much more sophisticated systems using magnetic fields and brain waves, to measure the internal skull pressure of infants with hydrocephalus ('water on the brain'), avoiding drilling into the skull.

Now we are exploring healthcare cybernetics that could transform surgery. At London's Imperial College, a virtual operating theatre allows students to practice in a realistic simulator, and new ways of linking surgeon and scalpel can 'pre-programme' delicate procedures, to avoid cutting vital nerves and vessels.

Devices to probe inside the body capture our imagination. Will we see miniature submarines manned by a tiny human crew, to navigate the body and investigate disease where and when it happens? Unlikely, but unmanned devices to do the same cannot be far off. We already have cameras to go pretty much anywhere in the body, to visualize abnormalities and guide surgeons. They may be uncomfortable to have inserted but they are a lot better than undergoing general surgery!

Devices can also be implanted to sense biochemical imbalance and deliver therapy in proportion to need. Insulin pumps (worn outside the body) detect the blood glucose level dropping and calculate the right infusion of insulin to correct it. Other combinations between drugs and delivery devices include drug-eluting stents (using cell growth inhibitors to help keep arteries open), implanted beads to control liver cancer, bone cements containing antibiotics and specialised dressings based on collagen for better wound healing.

Devices can also be geared to the body's electrical activity, and be reprogrammable as a patient's needs change, as with third generation 'cardioverter' defibrillators. Programmable electronic devices like this bring their own security challenges. Electronic security procedures like those that prevent wrongful access to your bank account can now be used to ensure only authorized personnel reprogramme your defibrillator!

There are practical problems of getting electrical power to implanted devices, but these problems actually become easier to solve as the devices get smaller. So-called 'piezo-electric nanogenerators' generate electrical power as the patient moves about: pressure changes charge up the tiny device, avoiding the need for a battery.

The brain—understanding it, training it, repairing it, enhancing it—will be the 'final frontier' for intelligent devices, as their function and that of the brain itself start to fuse together. This is probably not on our 20-year horizon, you may be relieved or disappointed to know!

In contrast, remote life signs monitoring is already here, thanks to the wireless revolution. Heart failure is the most common reason for hospital admissions in the US, costing $30 billion a year. Wearable monitors are now available to show heart rhythm, blood oxygen, etc., enabling health services to intervene before an event forces admission to hospital.

Nike shoes already track exercise and send the results to a mobile phone, and in the future to a health coach. Smart beds are doing the same with sleep patterns! With widespread mobile technology (four billion users already!), affordable broadband connectivity, smart phones and ingenious sensors the stage is set for an explosion in remote patient monitoring. This will revolutionize the management of diabetes, asthma, COPD, hypertension, Alzheimer's, obesity, and sleep disorders, as well as heart failure.

Jane's uncle **Dennis** had been on the medical watch list for some time. His sedentary lifestyle, as an accountant not given to much weekend sport, had made him overweight, his blood pressure was high despite taking anti-hypertensives (when he remembered), he had suffered deep vein thrombosis on a long-haul flight to his holiday in New Zealand and his doctors worried about the arrhythmia bouts he occasionally suffered.

Without some change in his life and without close supervision, his risk of a cardiac event before 65 was calculated as above 60%. At that level he more than qualified for the new LifeLine 24/7 device and the service that came with it. The device was an armband that simultaneously measured blood pressure, heart rate and blood glucose – these had been standard for some time. The new feature was an arrhythmia alert. This monitored the heart rhythm and sent a radio frequency signal to the monitoring service if anything other than a beat was skipped.

The service then called him on the special phone he always carried. That prompted him to immediately take the anti-arrhythmia drug he had been prescribed and advised him on how best to respond – sit down, breath deeply, go immediately to the hospital, depending on the severity of the attack.

It had already saved his life, his doctors estimated, more than once.

New medical practice—from craft industry to intelligent system

With every new medical technology comes the prospect of a new medical discipline. Sometimes this new discipline is accommodated, comfortably or less so, inside an established department of medicine. Radiology is one example— starting with X-ray examinations it has embraced other kinds of scans, and radiotherapy for cancer treatment. But sometimes the practice is so radically new that a whole new department of practice or a new pattern of treatment opens up. Minimally invasive surgery, organ transplants and molecular medicine are all recent examples. The more we create new branches of biomedical science the greater the number of clinical specialities we will produce.

What new disciplines might the next 20 years bring? Genomic medicine is an obvious candidate. Today we have genetic counselors, skilled in advising individuals and couples on the results of a relatively few common tests—for example for cystic fibrosis. But the number of genes associated in some way with disease is growing dramatically, so this field will undergo an enormous expansion.

When, for example, the genes for high colon cancer risk are fully known, patients can be tested for these early in their lives. Genomic specialists can then advise on when to start regular colonoscopy to check for polyps, whether to avoid all red meat, or balance with other forms of food intake, and whether to use fecal gene tests to spot the appearance of modified cells before they are seen in colonoscopy. This will create a whole new discipline.

Precision diagnostics will also change the definitions of disease, and so reshape specialties. Molecular tools to distinguish the different root causes of diabetes may result in patients being routed to different specialists, just as wider types and better quality of images already distinguish 'back pain' patients that would benefit most from orthopaedic surgery, neurosurgery or physiotherapy. The sharper the diagnosis the more specialised the medical practice will become. Diseases will be defined in terms of their molecular basis, not their symptoms.

Nanotechnology and intelligent devices will also open up a new discipline of programming and controlling them to achieve best effect in the body. The fusion of electrical engineering and clinical knowledge will produce a new breed of cyber-clinicians.

Patterns of care will change radically. In the place of 'trial and error' pathways, we will have greater precision, based on genetic or other types of profiling. Cross-checking with the outcomes of treatment options for other patients with similar profiles, will enable choice to be informed by thousands of personal experiences, not just the relatively few seen by the doctor who happens to be treating the patient.

The health informatics revolution will also enable us to rebalance the roles of specialists, family doctors, practice nurses, paramedics and pharmacists.

Much of the primary care that doctors deliver will come from other professionals, equipped with secure access to the patient's record and recommended pathways for diagnosis and treatment.

There is a real professional opportunity for pharmacists. They have most of the skills for long-term patient management and their walk-in high street locations make them convenient for patients, who trust their knowledge and discretion. They should train and equip themselves for an expanded role in the future of care.

The supply of new medical technology over the next 20 years will undoubtedly be breathtaking. But, like all technological progress through the centuries, it will also be unpredictable—for two reasons. First, it is often new technology that drives ideas, rather than the other way round. So when the first generation of technology appears it triggers refinements, new applications and new versions. These 'second generation' technologies then seek out the tougher problems they are equipped to solve. Second, the convergence of two different technologies often opens up completely new possibilities that the experts in each could never have guessed, just as MRI scans and keyhole surgery have done over the last two decades.

The next 20 years of healthcare will see the convergence of three dramatically different waves of invention—bioscience, information technology, and nano-technology. We are in for an exciting time!

However, each advance comes with a price tag. New drugs, cell therapies, imaging tools, informatics systems, and intelligent devices will all be more expensive than the technologies they replace. This is almost inevitable in any area of advance, as in cars, computers, and aircraft. What makes it a particular challenge in healthcare is fixed payer or government budgets and the difficulty that health systems have in phasing out the old to make way for the new.

If we cannot work out how to make new technology affordable to all the patients that could benefit, some would say it is unethical to develop it! Especially as demand for today's technology continues to rise rapidly, and health budgets with it, as we see in our next chapter.

Chapter 2

Healthcare demand—insatiable?

Demand for healthcare is unlike demand for anything else. Satisfying it simply increases future demand. This has always been so, but rightly this has so far not deterred us from meeting it. We constantly seek healthier and longer lives—or as a recent UK government report put it: 'adding years to life, and life to years'.

However, an important shift is underway in the expectations of health care consumers. Rather than expecting a few years of post-60s health, they expect to live in full vigour well into retirement. Indeed many want, or need to, stay active and alert enough to earn a living into their late 60s or even their 70s. This is in sharp contrast to their parents, most of whom expected to decline rapidly once they passed their 'three score years and ten'.

At the same time, the health of all—old and young—is threatened by self-inflicted tidal waves of obesity, smoking and alcoholism, and the chronic diseases they cause. On top of the diseases of abuse or physical decline we have the threat, indeed the certainty, of new diseases and new pandemics—often starting in the developing world but not staying there.

This is a powerful cocktail of what economists would call 'demand drivers'. Even without new and more costly technology, we face demands that will stretch and perhaps break the healthcare systems we built in the last century.

So, spending on health is set to continue to spiral. Europe spends an average of around 9.5% of Gross Domestic Product (GDP) on health, and this proportion has risen by about 1.5% over the last 10 years (Figure 2.1).

By 2009, the US was already at the 16% of GDP level. This is over $2 trillion, or $7,000 per person, per year. Growth in US health spending has somewhat slowed at around 7% per year, but remains about twice the rate of inflation, so could be over 20% of GDP, at over $4 trillion, by 2016. These are truly astounding numbers—driven by expectation, ageing, demands for universal access, escalating medical labour costs, chronic diseases, both self-inflicted and genetically determined, and diseases as yet unknown.

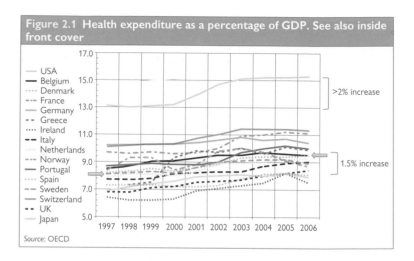

Figure 2.1 Health expenditure as a percentage of GDP. See also inside front cover

USA
Belgium
Denmark
France
Germany
Greece
Ireland
Italy
Netherlands
Norway
Portugal
Spain
Sweden
Switzerland
UK
Japan

>2% increase

1.5% increase

1997 1998 1999 2000 2001 2002 2003 2004 2005 2006

Source: OECD

Giving all citizens equity in access to care—the only course for a civilized society—can only drive demand still higher. The Obama plan comes with a price tag estimated by the Congressional Budget Office at $1.3 trillion (for an additional 16 million people covered) over the next 10 years. This adds further strain to already under-funded Medicare and Medicaid budgets (the unfunded Medicare liabilities are already estimated at $37 trillion!).

Let us examine each of these major demand drivers.

Great expectations—from passive patient to demanding consumer

When the UK's National Health System was first launched 60 years ago, the idea of comprehensive health care available free to all at the point of need was revolutionary. Before this, people either drained their savings to pay for treatment, or paid into employer-organized schemes insuring against serious illness. Or they suffered and died.

How people's expectations about their health have changed! Except in those countries where no insurance cover (state or private) exists, or for those individuals not covered by insurance, people in the developed world have come to expect either to receive most treatment for free, or to pay only a small proportion of the cost. But the greater change in expectations is in what people expect their healthcare to achieve. Not just rescue them from catastrophic illness – heart attacks, cancer, and the like. But also provide remedies for depression, obesity, impotence, and the aches and pains of old age. And rightly so. We now have the knowledge to keep people well, and give them fuller lives, not just try to rescue them at late stages of decline.

Expectations are nowhere higher than in the US. Patients demand the best, and often sue when they don't get it. This has driven defensive medicine – doctors running tests or providing treatment they do not believe to be necessary, just to minimize the risks of medical liability claims. A simple, true doctor's story tells it all:

> 'A recent complaint letter I received involved the cost of a chest pain workup in a healthy young woman. She presented with a one week history of substernal chest pressure and shortness of breath that were worse both on exertion and inspiration. She was a cigarette smoker who took no medications and had no family history of heart disease or premature death. She denied cough, fever, or leg pain. Her vital signs and examination were unrevealing. She was basically just young and healthy.

> After her ECG, chest X-ray, complete blood count, blood chemistries, and cardiac enzymes were reported as normal, I went back into the room and explained the rationale for CT scan of the chest (to rule out pulmonary embolism, primarily). She refused the test, and she was discharged against medical advice after I carefully documented our conversation, her awareness of the potential risks, and her acceptance of the risks of death or disability. After receiving her medical bills, she was shocked at the charges and filed a complaint with the patient relations department of our hospital. As an uninsured patient, her bill for my level 5 evaluation and management charge was $500. The addition of the ER facility fee, laboratory studies, X rays, and Radiologist's professional fee brought the total bill to almost $4,000 even without the CT scan of the chest (which would have probably added another $1,500 or so to her tab, I imagine).

> She claimed that she discussed her symptoms with a relative in Guatemala who is a physician, and he told her to take some ibuprofen, and of course she got better. Why didn't I think of that?

> If I was a physician in Guatemala, I wouldn't have ordered any tests either, and I would have only charged her a couple of chickens, or maybe a young goat. In America, unfortunately, we are required to overcharge, over-test, and over-document in order to keep the hyenas at bay.'

A recent US survey found that four out of five doctors said they ordered more tests than strictly necessary, and three-quarters said they made more referrals than they should, also for defensive reasons or because of other perverse incentives. Doctors' estimates of other doctors' defensive practices were higher still. Recent studies by both Mark McClelland (the former head of CMS, the US government's central health funding agency) and the accounting firm Price Waterhouse Coopers, suggest the total cost in the US is about 10% of total health spending.

As so often happens, a trend established in the US soon goes global, and defensive medicine is no exception.

With greater expectations also come greater legitimate treatment costs. When the NHS was launched, the doctor's medicine cabinet had penicillin, aspirin, paracetamol, diuretics, and little else. Now the UK national formulary has thousands of different medicines. And, of course, the number of diagnostic and surgical procedures has also risen dramatically. So our greater expectations can increasingly be met.

Patients are no longer passive and grateful recipients of whatever the system provides—they are consumers, with high standards. And none more than the generation now beginning to enter the years of physical decline and growing healthcare demand—the baby boomers.

The ageing of the baby boomers—from boom to bust

Ageing, someone once said, is better than the alternative—at least for individuals. But for whole societies, the major demographic shift underway—to have between a quarter and a third of people above 60—spells a level of demand for healthcare that is truly unprecedented. As healthcare improves it only sets itself greater challenges. This baby boomer generation will be the first for which a majority will live 15 to 20 years beyond retirement—a vigorous, useful life into their 70s, 80s, and even 90s.

It is not just countries like America and Britain that are 'greying' rapidly. The developing world is catching up fast, and the gap will close further as their economies develop and the basic needs of clean water, sanitation and adequate nutrition are met. Even the Chinese are worried, as their one child per family policy progressively shifts the balance between young and old, productive and dependent. So they are planning to allow two children to approved families. In some countries the problem is already acute: in Japan, 40% of the population will soon be over 65.

The most immediate impact this has on the affordability of healthcare is the so-called dependency ratio: the over 65s (largely on the receiving end of healthcare) versus those still in employment (paying for it). In Britain, as in most other developed nations, this ratio is steadily rising, at 1.2% each year.

Looking longer term, the baby boomers are actually a relatively small 'blip' on the rising age curve. Their children and grandchildren form two great waves of future healthcare demand!

So, over the next 20 years the good news that we are surviving longer will bring with it a huge expansion in healthcare demand. As the baby boomers reach the 70s and 80s, the degenerative diseases like arthritis and Alzheimer's will inevitably take hold. In a very real way, these will not be old people, at least in their own eyes: just old joints, or old hearts or old brains. As the basic health of our bodies improves, we will increasingly have the tragedy of physically fit people in their 60s–70s with advanced Alzheimer's, or of a

90 year-old with all her faculties but unable to move a muscle without severe arthritic pain.

Alzheimer's poses the greatest of all the ageing challenges ahead. Periodically, the UK pharmaceutical industry reviews the topics on which the public call for more medical research. The first and second priorities in the latest survey held no surprises—cancer and heart disease. But in the last few years a new, third priority has emerged—Alzheimer's, with most people saying much more research is needed.

The symptoms of advanced Alzheimer's—memory loss, repetitive, and even violent behaviour, and a draining away of personality—are deeply distressing for both the sufferer and their family. The changes in the brain that accompany these symptoms are 'tangles and plaques' of a rogue protein called beta-amyloid. These have so-far proved irreversible, but no-one knows whether they are the cause of the disease or simply the build-up of protein as a result of other changes. Much remains to be unraveled about the earlier stages of the disease.

It is estimated that there are about 700,000 Alzheimer's sufferers in the UK—only about 1% of the population, but one in 14 of those above 65 and a staggering one in six over 80. Because of the demographic trends, the total number of sufferers is set to more than double by the middle of the century. Unless we have an effective therapy—one of the pharmaceutical industry's greatest challenges—the strain on both the healthcare and social care systems will be enormous.

Cancer is also largely a disease of the ageing, despite the attention-grabbing cases of young relatives or celebrities struck down in their prime. It is in our 60s and 70s that cancer most often appears, but better diagnostic tools are enabling us to catch it earlier and earlier. Then begins a lengthy, usually multi-step process of therapy involving surgery, radiotherapy, and anti-cancer drugs. A single case can easily cost hundreds of thousands of dollars or pounds.

Less devastating and costly, but still a major burden on the patient and on the system, is osteoarthritis, a condition for which no effective treatment has yet been developed. Anti-inflammatory drugs can help, but still there is a steady increase in pain levels and loss of mobility and the ability to care for oneself, resulting in other burdens on the family and society.

Even if we can avoid these diseases, the frailty of old age means that long-term care—whether included in official health expenditures or not – will represent a growing burden. In developed countries this accounts for around 15% of health spending, even if most of it is borne by families rather than the state. It is better and cheaper for society for families to care for the elderly rather than place them in expensive institutions—although this is already the fate of one in 20 of those over 65. We can expect an expansion in state-supported and mandated 'national elderly care' insurance systems, as already seen in Germany, Holland, and Japan and under intense discussion in the UK.

The challenge of access—coverage and equality

The scandal of more than 40 million US citizens without health insurance has finally reached the top of the political agenda in the US. Universal coverage is now on the horizon, the main debate now being how to achieve it affordably.

In the short term this costs money, a great deal of it, as Massachusetts discovered implementing its own universal coverage plan. In the three years since launching the plan, costs rose 42%, an increase of $600 million, as a result of covering an additional 432,000 people. This has caused the state government to experiment with systems to drive better management of chronic disease rather than reward the sheer quantity of care provided. But policymakers there are also threatening to cap insurance premiums and hospital fees and to limit coverage to care that passes tests of comparative clinical or cost effectiveness. Overall, a tough prescription for the state with more doctors per capita than any other, and with some of the most sophisticated and therefore expensive academic medical centres.

As the implications of Obama's healthcare reform sink in across America, other states are counting the cost of extra coverage. The bill for California alone is estimated at more than $500 million a year in extra funding for the Medicaid programme.

In the long run, of course, universal coverage of primary care will avoid many of the expensive late stage interventions that health systems often pay for anyway. Massachusetts estimated a $250 million saving in emergency care for the uninsured. But it takes some years to see this payback on the initial massive investment.

The US is far from being the only nation with a healthcare access problem. Adequate access exists only when individuals can access and benefit from healthcare services, either free or affordable at the point of need, without barriers of race or culture. Even in the so-called universal coverage systems in much of Europe, there are populations that have inadequate access. In some cases this is because of their remote location. In others because there are too few doctors, or too few that speak the same language and share the same culture. Or insufficient specialists in a key area, such as cancer care in the UK. Any of these can be barriers to access.

Fully closing the access gap will drive costs still higher for all systems, if we meet the expanded needs no more efficiently than we do today.

Obesity—and other self-inflicted wounds

Of all the health issues that cast a shadow over the future of the 21st century health system, the dual threats of obesity and diabetes loom largest. Ample food, habitual meat- and sugar-rich diets, less exercise: all drive unhealthy weight gain. And then, as a result, for many comes Type II diabetes—some years behind obesity, but with steady step.

Media stories and dramatic statistics on obesity abound. Ironically, pictures of the morbidly obese may actually desensitize some people to their own situation. Assailed by images of the grossly obese, people that are just plain overweight fail to see their weight as a real problem. As we might expect, women tend to pay more attention to weight, but men underestimate the problem. 'Middle-age spread' now often makes its appearance long before middle age, as a scan of most football stadiums will confirm. As someone put it: 'football is a game in which 22 people in need of rest are watched by 50,000 people in need of exercise'.

It is because obesity increases the risk of Type II diabetes that we should be so concerned. It is estimated that 24 million in the US have diabetes, and 57 million more have 'pre-diabetes', a syndrome that increases the risk of the full-blown disease by five to six times.

The total annual economic cost of diabetes in the US in 2007 was estimated to be $174 billion—of which medical expenditures totalled $116 billion ($6,650 a year for each person—half of it for complications). Indirect costs—resulting from increased absenteeism, reduced productivity, disease-related unemployment disability, and loss of productive capacity due to early mortality—totalled $58 billion. One out of every five health care dollars in the US is spent caring for someone with diagnosed diabetes.

This is not just an American problem. It was recently estimated that one in five UK hospital patients suffers from diabetes.

It is the long-term complications of uncontrolled diabetes that are most worrying—for the patient and health system alike. Peripheral neuropathy—death of nerve-endings in the extremities—leads to foot ulcers that heal slowly, or not at all. This can ultimately result in gangrene and amputations. Diabetic macular oedema, leading ultimately to blindness, is a second serious complication. But the biggest diabetes 'demand multiplier' of all is cardiovascular disease—requiring anything from vascular surgery for the legs to cardiac bypass surgery or transplant operations.

Despite all the media attention and public health warnings, obesity and diabetes continue their upward trend, and economic downturns can actually aggravate the problem as they worsen diets.

Smoking remains one of the most devastating of the world's avoidable health problems, and is still on the rise in fast-developing parts of the world. Links to lung cancer are well established but still not well enough registered in the teenage mind to stop millions of young people starting a habit that is one of the hardest to stop. Young women seem to be particularly vulnerable, despite advertising bans, pack warnings, and health education—they seem immune to anything the adult world can devise.

COPD (chronic obstructive pulmonary disease) is lung cancer's much less publicized cousin, although not exclusively caused by smoking. Only one in five smokers develop it: other causes are occupational exposures, asthma, and air pollution. There is mounting evidence that it is not one disease but several, with genetic variations playing their part. With one in 20 Americans affected, there are more than 13 million sufferers in the US, all at risk of debilitating breathlessness and emergency admissions to hospital.

While smoking has begun to decline in many developed countries, alcoholism is firmly on the rise. Of the liver transplants done in the UK since 2000, alcoholism was the largest cause, followed by hepatitis (also now largely preventable). As well as liver failure, excess alcohol also leads to depression and heart failure and damage to the nervous system.

Drunkenness has been a social problem since biblical times—so what is new? In short, easier access to cheap alcohol at earlier and earlier ages. Teenagers that start drinking at ages 14 or younger greatly increase their chances of a lifelong drink problem. I recently sat behind two teenage girls on a train travelling into London in the early evening. They were passing a wine bottle between them and excitedly talking of getting 'smashed' that evening, regarding getting an early start as an advantage in a competition of sorts. Of course, many teenagers leave this behind with other teenage excesses, but if they are unlucky enough to have the wrong genetic make-up combined with less self-control they will be unable to do this, and early recklessness could blight the rest of their lives.

The impact of alcohol and alcoholism on the economy is huge. In 2000 the US National Institute on Alcohol Abuse and Alcoholism estimated a national bill of $185 billion, with the costs in lost current and future earnings, and those from automobile accidents and fires dwarfing direct medical costs. If other substance abuse is added, the total rises to $300 billion, a number to rival the cost of bank bailouts!

Alcoholism is, of course, not a purely health problem with purely health solutions. Integrated strategies are needed, embracing social workers, police, and voluntary sector agencies. But even with these measures, the burden of health issues from alcohol abuse seems destined to rise further in the years ahead.

Chronic disease, caused or accelerated by lifestyle choices, must be a major focus when we are designing healthcare in 2030. In the US, one-third of the 18–34 age group, two-thirds of those between 45 and 64, and 90% of the elderly already suffer from a chronic condition. The five biggest chronic diseases—diabetes, congestive heart failure, coronary artery disease, asthma/COPD, and depression account for most of the burden, and all these problems are increasing in most parts of the world. Unless we tackle them more effectively, they will overwhelm us.

George's cousin **Alan** drank like a fish. And, unlike fish, not just water. First, it was just a matter of comment and jokes from the rest of the family. But, by his mid-40s, there were unmistakable signs of liver cirrhosis. His liver enzymes were off the charts, and he frequently felt the tell-tale soreness under his right ribcage.

Alan finally joined Alcoholics Anonymous. His wife painfully poured the remaining contents of the cocktail cabinet down the sink. But the abdominal scans were clear—without a new liver he was unlikely to last long, despite being only in his late 40s.

There were two treatment options, both expensive. After tissue typing he was told that a transplant was uncertain. The more likely option required taking his bone marrow cells, transforming these into pluripotent stem cells and then into liver cells. These were then grown within a biocompatible framework into an artificial liver, which would then be implanted alongside what was left of his own. It was a six-hour operation that required a full surgical team. When the costs of this were added to those of the process to create the new liver, and the drugs needed to stabilise it, the total was well over $100,000.

Since this was regarded as an avoidable condition the copayment terms from his health plan were onerous.

The cost of new technology—becoming unaffordable

Although it is not the cost of new treatments that will bankrupt healthcare, in the short run they clearly add to the problem. New technology is often layered over old, rather than replacing it. But even when the old is displaced the new is more expensive, at levels beyond the level of general inflation. The UK's Department of Health routinely assumes a steady growth of 1 to 1.5% per annum in the health budget from the arrival of new technology.

At its root the problem is the spiralling cost of development, resulting from ever-tighter regulation. These higher R&D expenses in turn demand higher prices, in order to earn adequate returns on investment.

Rigorous drug regulation began in earnest with thalidomide. Prescribed as a sleeping pill, the drug resulted in the birth of thousands of babies with serious birth defects. As a result of the rigorous testing introduced in the years that followed, such an event is unthinkable today. All new drugs are screened for harmful teratogenic (foetal development) effects; this screen is now but one of a wide range of tests to minimize the risks of new medicines causing heart problems, liver or kidney disease or other 'off-target' effects for which predictive tests exist.

Each new 'serious adverse event' caused by new drugs adds to the burden of testing for all those that follow. This results in mounting numbers and costs of both pre-clinical (i.e. laboratory-based) testing and also the complexity, length and costs of human clinical trials. The rarer the adverse event, the larger the number of patients needed to detect them in clinical trials.

Tougher testing also multiplies the risk of a medicine being rejected – either by the company investigating the drug or by the regulator (the FDA in the Unites States, the EMA in Europe) that controls the entry of new medicines to the market. The dramatically high failure rate in potential new medicines in turn multiplies the average cost for each new successful medicine.

Regulation of the clinical trials themselves, though well meaning, is getting out of hand. In its current form, Good Clinical Practice (GCP) dictates that every trial collects all 'Serious Adverse Events' (SAEs) whether or not they are truly drug-related (as opposed to being the result of the disease itself). All results are then reported to all investigators on the trial, all ethics committees involved and all Data Monitoring Committees. The result is an avalanche of paperwork that everyone is supposed to study and few actually do. One recent trial of 20,000 people was estimated to spend $12m on this step alone.

As one clinician has put it, all patients with a disease represent an 'adverse event', and side-effects of medicines need to be put in proportion to unmet medical need.

The current rigid, costly, multi-stage process is shown in Figure 2.2.

Regulators are in a tough position, particularly in the US, where their decisions are frequently drawn into political controversy. Their job is to establish the relationship between benefit and risk for a new medicine. However, they get none of the credit for the benefit and much of the blame for the risks that might result from release of a new drug with dangerous side-effects, or a device that malfunctions.

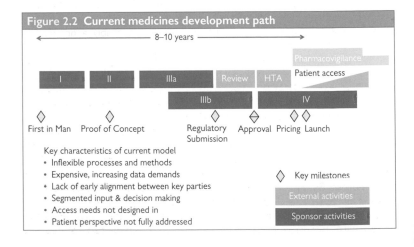

Figure 2.2 **Current medicines development path**

The resulting trend in the cost of new medicines and technologies is completely unsustainable. For new medicines in 2001 it was estimated to be $800 million per new drug; by 2003 it had risen to $900 million; most recently it was calculated as $1.3–1.7 billion. If we were to extrapolate this cost spiral at an extra $100 million a year, each new drug in 20 years' time will cost over $3.5 billion. The choice is clear: either we forget new technology and satisfy ourselves with what we have today, or we must redesign the process.

The peril of pandemics—crossing species and crossing borders

Throughout human history, pandemics of disease have swept around the globe and decimated populations. The Black Death or Great Plague of the 1300s fundamentally reshaped Europe, with between a third and two-thirds of the inhabitants of cities, towns and villages dying. The global population reduced by about 75 million.

The most likely source of the disease was rodents in central Asia, and the disease was then carried eastward by the Mongol tribes and westward through the Crimea to Sicily, and from there on to almost every part of Europe, already weakened by food shortages and harsh winters. This outbreak was not an isolated one and bubonic plague returned to Europe in almost every generation until the 1700s.

Most of those who survived multiple attacks of the plague probably did so because they had a different genetic profile yielding a stronger immune system. So the disease was a major force in determining today's genetic pool. The result is a hyperactive immune system that probably results in higher levels of asthma and similar immune disorders.

The most recent devastating pandemic was the 1918 'Spanish' flu outbreak, overshadowed by the First World War, whose troop movements was probably a major factor in its spread. Again it was probably a non-human origin, most likely from birds.

The influenza virus contains two proteins, hemagglutinin (H) and neuraminidase (N), and different versions of the virus are distinguished by a numbering system HXNY. The two proteins have important roles in infection: the 'H' enables the virus to bind to the human cell, and the 'N' to escape from the cell once the virus has multiplied inside it.

The flu pandemic in 1918 was H1N1, and this type made a dramatic reappearance in the 2009 'swine flu', containing gene fragments from swine, avian and human influenza A viruses. Fortunately the discovery of NAI antivirals (neuraminidase inhibitors) gives the human race some level of preparedness. But we also know that the virus evolves to escape anti-viral attack if it is active in enough humans for a sufficient length of time.

Other flu strains are hovering in the background—the avian flu H5N1 caused alarm two years earlier, when it appeared in various parts of Asia. All this suggests that a true pandemic on the scale of the Spanish flu of 1918 is a matter of time, and we must have the right preparations in place.

A special case of the threat of global infections is the spectre of bioterrorism. Fourteen anthrax-laden letters sent in 2001 in the US that caused just five deaths put both the nation and the world on bioterrorism alert, and triggered billions in biodefence investment. One beneficial result from the threat has been the development of faster detection and confirmation tests for rare infections, and software that picks up an emerging pandemic from routine health reports.

Jane recalled the 2027 pandemic of H9N1 influenza. The world had little immunity to this strain, which had picked up both swine and bird flu genetic material in its passage through species. There had not been a virus quite like it in living memory—and therefore was unknown to the 'immune' memory of most of the world's ten billion people.

The new threat emerged from Indonesia, but public health officials in Singapore where passengers from Jakarta began to arrive with fever, were the first to spot the problem. And then 'spikes' of infection appeared in the 'global health surveillance system' in Hong Kong and Malaysia, in families of those who had just arrived from Indonesia.

Based on its genetic profile, scientists had estimated that the fatality rate from this highly virulent strain could be over one in 10. Fortunately, the world had stockpiled a broad spectrum influenza vaccine that would give some immunity, but as soon as the new strain emerged, a worldwide race began to create a strain-specific vaccine. The programme broke all records, using the cell-based development and production method that had long since displaced the growing of vaccine in hen's eggs. From the first strain arriving in the laboratory to production at scale took less than four months.

With the learning from the two earlier pandemics (H1N1 in 2009 and H5N1 in 2015) the world had negotiated its way through all the complex political and health issues that pandemics pose. How does a poorer country in which it first arises ensure that they have affordable access to vaccine, without slowing down the global sharing of samples and full-scale health surveillance collaboration? With most of the production facilities concentrated in a few rich countries, how to avoid politically driven national selfishness? How to ensure that international quarantine roles are sensibly applied to contain the pandemic while vaccine is developed?

All these questions had been the subject of intense international negotiation in the 2010s, with the World Health Organization given real authority to coordinate the world's response. Even so, Jane remembered with a tear, her cousin Terry was on business in Singapore in 2027, succumbed to the virus in the first two weeks, and—despite anti-virals and intensive care—was one of the two hundred thousand people who died. But without the world's determination to act together against viral infections the toll would have been hundreds of millions.

The real problem with infectious disease is that it so easily crosses borders, both national borders and the borders between species. Close encounters between man and cohabitants of the planet create most of our pandemics. Mosquitoes bring us malaria. Birds fly in with avian flu or West Nile virus. Intensively farmed pigs develop a newly virulent strain of flu. Ticks from deer bestow Lyme disease. Eating infected beef gives us a human version of 'mad cow' disease. Better animal husbandry can bring human benefits, but cannot prevent all pandemics.

The most probable culprit for HIV is the simian monkey. It is estimated that the virus crossed into man in Africa about a century ago, perhaps through a monkey bite. It seems to have appeared in Haiti in the mid-60s, and crossed to the US around 1970. It was then in the early 1980s that promiscuous sex and needle sharing among drug addicts spread the human virus, first in San Francisco and then throughout the world.

HIV is the most devastating global pandemic since the Plague. There are now 33 million known cases; 2.5 million are newly diagnosed and more than 2 million die each year. The virus has wrought havoc with lives, families, health systems, and economies. There are more than 15 million AIDS orphans in sub-Saharan Africa. The cost of adequately treating this global pandemic is estimated at $25 billion a year, far in excess of the current level of resources devoted to the problem. Even to treat patients in the rich, developed world requires continuous advance in pharmaceutical discovery to keep pace with the virus as it evolves to evade therapy.

Ultimately, we cannot treat our way out of this pandemic: our twin hopes for a lasting solution are prevention and vaccination. But developing an HIV vaccine is proving the toughest challenge that has ever faced vaccine researchers. The last few years have seen 'three steps forward, two steps back', although the promising results from a 2009 Thailand trial seem a step forward.

HIV lowers the body's resistance to infection. So it is often accompanied, particularly in the developing world, by tuberculosis. Many HIV-infected patients actually die of TB, which itself is developing in worrying ways. The emergence and spread of strains extremely resistant to the current complicated drug regimen is now as much a threat to the developed as to the developing world. So not only are TB cases arising in major cities of the Western world, they are frequently very tough to treat.

The third horseman of the pandemic apocalypse is malaria. Very widespread across the developing South, with the long-term threat that global warming will extend its reach northwards. Newer drugs, like Coartem, are quite effective, but in many parts of the world patients are receiving cheap but ineffective medicines that simply spread drug resistance further. So, while research into new treatments continues, via the successful public-private partnership, Medicines for Malaria, the greatest long term hope is an effective vaccine.

The costs of combating the combined global epidemics of HIV/AIDS, malaria, and TB are truly staggering. The US government's PEPFAR programme (the President's Emergency Plan for AIDS Relief) has as its goal preventing 12 million HIV cases, treating 2 million people and supporting 12 million others. Along with $4 billion for TB and $5 billion for malaria, the total 5-year bill is around $50 billion! And that leaves at least 20 million other HIV-positive cases for other HIV funders to reach. If there is any good news, it is that HIV prevalence is now beginning to level off.

These diseases, now all too familiar to us, face future competition. Margaret Chan, the Director General of the World Health Organization, recently wrote that new infectious diseases are emerging at the historically unprecedented rate of one per year. And 2 billion air passenger journeys per year ensure they spread across the globe in hours, not the three years it took the Black Death to make its way from Asia into every corner of Europe.

Epidemics can be fearsomely expensive even when they are well contained. The SARS epidemic of 2003 was serious, but a speedy combination of primary care, screening and travel restrictions brought the outbreak under control within a few months. Only 8,400 people were infected. But the economic cost was staggering—an estimated $60 billion.

As we saw in the 2009 swine flu outbreak, a pandemic can originate almost anywhere on the globe—this time in Mexico. While the fatality level has been low, the need to gear up the prevention, vaccination and treatment machine across the world cost billions—not to mention the economic impact of other measures such as travel restrictions, the culling of animals and the closure of markets.

This is probably a good point to stop listing dangerous pandemics! We could go on to look at dengue fever, West Nile virus, or the dreaded Ebola. The point is that we can unfortunately expect nature to constantly produce new pandemic challenges, and for the pathogens we already have to evolve and so evade drug therapy. Pandemic-driven healthcare demands and costs will remain a looming reality for the foreseeable future.

Developing world demands—the ultimate healthcare challenge

Most pandemics make their greatest impact in the developing world, because of the lower level of public health and basic care available. But these gaps in health systems also result in growing burdens of untreated non-infectious disease, as diet and lifestyles change.

In recent years the developed world has awoken to the tremendous level of global health inequalities. Well-meaning resolutions have been passed to make healthcare a human right—but meaningless unless governments in both the developed and developing world make these rights their responsibilities. Of the eight ambitious Millennium Development Goals, three are directly health-related—reduce child mortality (by two-thirds in children under five), improve maternal health (reducing death in childbirth by three-quarters and achieving universal access to reproductive health), and combat HIV/AIDS, malaria and other diseases.

If we are to reach these goals, we need to redouble our efforts, and this costs money, even if many of the challenges can be met with quite basic care. (Only a half of developing world births take place with a birth attendant, for example.) Wherever we look there are needs: insufficient doctors and medical auxiliaries; inadequate facilities and medical equipment; non-existent supply chains needed to take even cheap generic medicines to rural areas.

To rise to the challenge, several developed countries (especially the US, the UK, the Netherlands, and Norway) have health budgets not just for themselves but for parts of the developing world. However, the greatest generosity has come from just one family. The Bill and Melinda Gates Foundation devotes the majority of the Microsoft founder's personal fortune to tackling developing world health, funding most of the efforts to find new drugs for malaria and TB via the two leading drug PDPs (Product Development Partnerships)—Medicines for Malaria and the TB Alliance. Both PDPs are working with academic researchers, medical charities and pharmaceutical companies to create a pipeline of new medicines for these two scourges. Neither disease has a developed world market large enough to drive normal economically-oriented R&D investment.

Developing world health demands call urgently for the resources of the Western nations. Although they typically come from the international development budgets rather than health, they still affect the staff and financial resources available to meet local needs. Ignoring them is not an option.

Even without these extra costs of attacking developing world health problems, the higher expectations of ageing Western populations facing the assaults of lifestyle diseases and periodic pandemics spells a rate of demand growth certain to outstrip the growth of our economies. This is not a temporary problem: it is an unavoidable part of our future. Let us turn to the consequences of runaway demand meeting ever-costlier supply.

Chapter 3

Medical meltdown—unavoidable?

As we combine the dual pressures of new technology supply with the remorseless growth in demand, we seem to face an unaffordable healthcare future.

We can already see the early signs. Until recently most economies grew strongly, but their healthcare budgets grew even faster. Health insurance costs in the US have risen by over 70% since 2000. Over the same period, average total health spending as a share of GDP in the major European countries increased from about 8% to around 9.5%.

Yet, access to the best that medical technology can provide remains very unequal. The more than 40 million who are uninsured in America have yet to experience 21st century healthcare. And rationing of expensive newer treatments in Britain has caused pain to patients and embarrassment to politicians.

Until recently the backdrop in both cases has at least been healthy economic growth. The recent recession reminds us that there is no guarantee of growth, and now healthcare budgets will be squeezed with all others, with the newest health technologies often bearing the brunt of the squeeze.

So, as both the supply of ever-more expensive technology and the need and expectation for healthcare increase, are we doomed to see a medical meltdown? Let's do some very rough calculations of the impact of the supply and demand trends. Most advanced (OECD) countries have seen their health expenditures grow steadily in real terms over the last 10 years, at annual rates averaging between 2.5 and 5%.

Layer on to this the likely impact of the accelerating ageing of the population (say 1%), and the greater expectation level of these better informed, more demanding baby boomers (say 1–2%).

Add in the result of the greater levels of obesity, diabetes and alcohol abuse in the next generations coming through (say another 1%). If we combine these demand forces with the higher costs of the new medicines and technologies emerging from R&D laboratories around the world (1–2%), then we can expect the bill for the healthcare we ideally need to rise at between 6 and 9% in real terms each year.

Slide of percentages

No-one expects economic growth in countries like the US and UK to keep pace with this. Even if we take the lower figure of 5%, over a 20-year period this will result in real healthcare costs two and a half times those we fund today.

Of course, we could simply accept this health budget growth as inevitable and divert funds from other public and private budgets to meet it. However, we have only to look at the fierce US reaction to costly ObamaCare, and to the current clampdown on the UK's NHS budget to realize this is very unlikely.

In this era of a growing gap between the healthcare we want and the healthcare we can afford, the consequence of failing to bring healthcare costs under control will be doubly dire. We will neither be able to bring the exciting new technology we described in Chapter 1 into routine use in patient care, nor satisfy the demand laid out in Chapter 2 for today's level of care for an ageing, more demanding population. That is what 'meltdown' would mean in practice.

We have three options to tackle the problem. The first is to lower expectations, and tell people to be satisfied with what is on offer now, and with their allotted span of 'three score years and ten'. (Or of course, following Aldous Huxley, euthanize them at the appointed hour!)

The second option is the one most European governments have opted for: controlling supply, by rationing access to costly care and applying a challenging cost-effectiveness threshold for any new treatments. Bodies like NICE, in England, the Transparency Commission in France and IQWG in Germany, constantly assess new health technologies and pronounce them cost-effective, or—very often—not, at least not at prices set by their innovators.

Over the long term neither of these options is sustainable. In no other walk of life do we either tell people to be satisfied with what they have, or demand every innovation prove its cost-effectiveness before it is released. Imagine telling people to be happy with the TVs or cell phones that exist today, or applying a strict governmental cost-effectiveness test to a new sports car or household appliance!

The reason, of course, why we do this in healthcare is that the patient, the consumer, neither pays out of her own pocket, nor exercises choice in the normal market sense. An insurer—either public or private—pays on their behalf out of a fixed budget. So, ultimately, they believe they must tell the patient what is available and so what their expectations can be.

This leaves us with the third and the only viable long-term option: to proactively tackle demand growth, make new technology more affordable and turn the patient into a consumer, making informed choices and actively participating in the funding equation. We must also make unprecedented strides in healthcare productivity, to close the gap between a fast-rising healthcare spending curve and what our society can afford.

Healthcare productivity—the outcomes achieved divided by the resources consumed—can be transformed by using 10 powerful levers: (1) focusing on

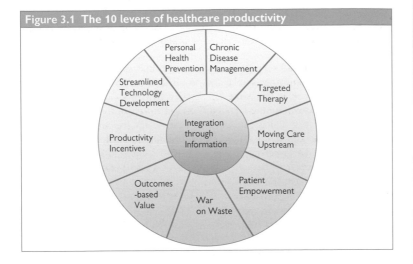

Figure 3.1 The 10 levers of healthcare productivity

Personal Health Prevention
Chronic Disease Management
Streamlined Technology Development
Targeted Therapy
Integration through Information
Productivity Incentives
Moving Care Upstream
Outcomes-based Value
Patient Empowerment
War on Waste

personalized prevention, (2) managing chronic disease with the power of process thinking, (3) radically streamlining new treatment development, (4) more intelligent targeting of care, (5) making war on waste, (6) empowering the patient, (7) valuing treatment choices on their outcomes, (8) moving care upstream, towards the patient and the community, (9) aligning everyone's incentives to drive productivity, and (10) harnessing the power of information to integrate the system around the patient.

If we use all of these levers shown in Figure 3.1 we will slow or stop many of the underlying drivers of health expenditure. What will be left will be the unavoidable cost of giving the right patient the right treatment, or preventive action, at the right time.

Let us examine each of these levers in turn, their value and how they could transform care by 2030.

Focus on prevention—from public health to personal programmes

A focus on prevention is the place to start for two reasons. Firstly, prevention is usually more cost-effective than cure. Secondly, it challenges the basic mindset of all health systems—that they are there to deal with disease. To be *ill-health* systems, in fact.

Let's start with this second point. It underlies so many aspects of healthcare. Politicians equate healthcare with hospitals. Doctors, most of whom will practice in the community, train there. Whether the local hospital stays open, and has an emergency department, is a touchstone for the general public. Professional language—from the 'chief complaint' for a visit to the accusation that the patient is just one of the 'worried well'—assumes the system is there to address the problems of the genuinely ill, not keep people well.

This is despite prevention having had the greatest impact on life expectancy—clean water, better sanitation, and smoking cessation have probably had more effect on lifespan than all the efforts of the medical profession!

The battle to improve life expectancy and quality of life via prevention strategies has never been more urgent. The life expectancy of a US citizen born in 1900 was 47; today it is 75 for men and 80 for women, with the greatest improvement in the poorer population. But in some parts of the country it has now begun to fall. In fact life expectancy fell or ceased to improve for 4% of American men and 19% of women over the 1990s, mainly in the southern states. Why? Mainly diseases linked to past smoking habits and to obesity.

The first is somewhat surprising until we remember that it was not until after the Second World War that women began to smoke as heavily as men, particularly among the poor. Here we might expect some future improvement, since both sexes have now started to quit in large numbers. However, obesity-driven disease is still very much on the rise. No less than 22 of the 50 US states now have more than a quarter of their populations obese. Deep fried food seems destined to reverse many of the health gains of the last century.

So the first thing to do is the obvious—target the major avoidable threats to health: smoking and poor diet.

Making smoking uncool, breaking the psychological link with the teenage goals of apparent maturity and toughness, should remain a top public health priority worldwide.

In contrast to smoking to appear mature, eating to become obese is certainly not a goal, for teenagers or for anyone else, except perhaps Sumo wrestlers. But it is almost as hard to leave behind, despite the mounting evidence of future health problems, such as heart disease, stroke, diabetes, some cancers, gout, and gallbladder disease. Being overweight can also aggravate problems such as sleep apnoea (interrupted breathing during sleep) and osteoarthritis (wearing away of the joints).

Just as with smoking, obesity's worst effects are seen many years after the behaviour that causes them. We need to use our increasingly sophisticated 'virtual world' technology to show people their futures if their life courses do not change. Seeing ourselves age with pain and disease will have more impact than today's 'don't do this, you'll regret it' messages. This is especially true for children, addicted to both the internet and to junk food: we should use the first addiction to attack the second.

Smoking and obesity, though hard to crack, are at least obvious to their sufferers. Many other diseases start invisibly and silently. One example is colon cancer. If it is caught, typically as a result of a colonoscopy, at its initial stage, surgery has a 95% success rate. But the disease often proceeds without symptom to later stages with much less hopeful prognoses. As we learn more about the connection between our genetic profiles and disease, we will be able to identify those most likely to suffer from the disease. We will combine dietary changes to prevent its development with more frequent scans to check we are being successful.

Early detection of many common cancers will join the predictive menu, as we learn more about their genetic basis. In the past, rigorous screening was seen as of doubtful value, as the 'number needed to treat' was high (the large number of people you would need to screen to find a genuine case). The extra worry caused to people who receive false positive results and hence are subjected to unnecessary stress, and the costs of the tests themselves, were also inhibitors. Greater precision and lower costs will change this equation.

The technology for some genetically-programmed personal prevention is already here. Craig Venter, the co-discoverer of the human genome sequence, used his own genome as the target and discovered he was predisposed to heart disease—so started taking a statin drug to lower his blood lipids. Incidentally, he also found that he had both copies of a gene for rapid caffeine metabolism, so his heart rhythms are unaffected by quadruple expressos! (Those without such gene variants can get jittery after a single cup of coffee.)

Prevention must also take care of bones and joints as we age. A startling number of people in their 50s and 60s develop back problems—often at a time in their lives in which they are healthy in most other ways. Our parents' problems are often an indication of what may lie ahead for us, and preventative exercise regimes, unexciting as they may be, are a lot more appealing than lengthy periods of pain and permanent weakness.

Conventional wisdom says that little can be done to reverse the one-way decline of vigour in otherwise healthy elderly people. But research has found that not only can regular exercise restore muscle function to near-youthful levels, but the underlying biochemistry is also renewed. Studies of the mitochondria (the cell's powerhouse) in old muscles showed that modest but regular exercise restored youthful patterns of gene expression! So 'use it or lose it' will be part of the answer.

The predictive tools for personal health will be arriving in the next decade. To combat the growth in preventable disease each person should be given the human equivalent of a preventive maintenance schedule, based on these tests and their family history. Adherence to this schedule should carry incentives, to ensure that action is not left too late.

The economic stakes are high. Preventing chronic disease saves substantial lifetime medical costs: two US examples—control of high blood pressure saves $13,700, and prevention of diabetes $34,500 per patient.

Excellent - Pt Examination 2030

No-one looks forward to the visit to a doctor. But, by the time **George** reached his 55th birthday, the five-year 'major body service' had become a very slick procedure that was mainly at the hands of medical technicians. 'Blood Work' was still a requirement, since it gave a clear readout on the functions of liver, pancreas, and kidneys. But much of the former 'prodding and probing' had been replaced by the full body MRI that could be compared with previous scans and taken to high resolution for specific organs like the brain and the prostate (George certainly did not miss the old digital rectal prostate exam). Eye and ear tests were now fully automated, to give the first signs of glaucoma, retinal detachment or loss of inner ear sensitivity.

Body fat measurement had become very sophisticated. The patient was presented with a 'total fat scan', showing its distribution through the body, and converting this, in combination with other measures like LDL—and HDL—cholesterol and homocysteine from the blood tests into quite accurate estimates for the probability of diabetes, coronary artery disease, stroke and other cardiovascular or metabolic disorders. Even greater accuracy came from combining these measures with the predisposition indices from George's gene sequence, done when he was 50. At that point the sequence gave him very broad indications on only a few preventable diseases. But the gene sequencing and advisory service had retained the results and regular updates were made to George's 'genetic probability files' as a result of new gene function discoveries or epidemiological studies.

George's '55-year service' had only a couple of potential problems on the horizon: a below-par kidney as a result of an infection two years earlier, and a 25% chance of type 2 diabetes by age 65. However, 55 was also the first really detailed look at his colon. Without any genetic indication of familial polypolyposis (multiple pre-cancerous growths in the colon) at 50 he had needed only a genetic test to detect cancerous cells in the stool. That had been negative, but now it was time to take a direct look!

How colonoscopy had changed! A simple chemical laxative had replaced the pints of unappetizing fluid he had seen his own parents swallow with a grimace. And the intelligent colonoscope plotted its own route through his insides, pausing only to photograph and biopsy any suspicious irregularities, for the doctor's later perusal. Not wanting to watch its progress, George had enjoyed a virtual reality flight over the Fijian islands in the slightly high and happy state of mind brought on by the sedatives and relaxants still used to avoid discomfort.

As knowledge of the links between genes, diet and lifestyle accumulates, our personal health future can be painted more accurately and our prevention plan woven into the fabric of our lives. Preventable and postponable disease will come under greater control.

Management of chronic disease—with the power of process thinking

Despite all our efforts at prevention, better management of chronic disease must remain a top priority. Once developed, diseases like diabetes, heart disease, arthritis, osteoporosis—worsening when untreated to the point that expensive 'rescue operations' are needed—will still be major drivers of health demand.

It is estimated that 133 million Americans, 45% of the population, suffer from some form of chronic disease and that this accounts, one way or another, for 75% of healthcare costs. So managing patients with such diseases is central to affordable healthcare.

Type II diabetes is a classic in this respect. It may have its onset in the 40s, but—if poorly controlled—will result in foot ulcers, worsening eyesight, heart problems and more, until in their 50s, 60s, and 70s patients may face amputations, blindness and heart attacks. And it was recently estimated by the RAND Corporation that diabetics in the US receive less than half the preventative care that could avoid or delay these serious consequences. These include simple and cheap remedies, like beta-blockers to lower high blood pressure and aspirin to avoid clotting.

Rose, George's mother, was now nearly 80. Like her own mother before her, she was quite slight in build, frail even, but also still quite active. A bone density scan in her 60s showed that she had already lost quite a bit of bone mass and so she received the annual vaccination that slowed the course of the osteoporosis. This worked quite well for some time, but the regular bone resorption tests that came with her check-up had started to show the problem reoccurring. At this rate, a heavy fall would give her a broken hip, or worse.

Her specialist put her on a personal bone recovery and joint strengthening plan. This involved a high calcium diet, low on meat, and a course of a new drug that actually reversed the course of the disease by rebinding the calcium into the bone. Also she had a daily exercise programme, since it had been discovered that even mild regular exercise rebuilt the muscles that supported the joints, even in those previously thought to be too old for the gym.

In the UK, chronic disease is estimated to account for 80% of primary care doctors' visits and over 60% of hospital bed-days. Type II diabetes alone accounts for nearly 5% of NHS costs, half of it spent on inpatient care, for complications such as amputation, stroke, ischaemic heart disease, heart failure, and blindness. People with diabetes are admitted to hospital twice as often and stay twice as long. In sharp contrast to these costly inpatient events, preventive medication accounts for only 2% of treatment costs.

Figure 3.2 Chronic disease patient management flow

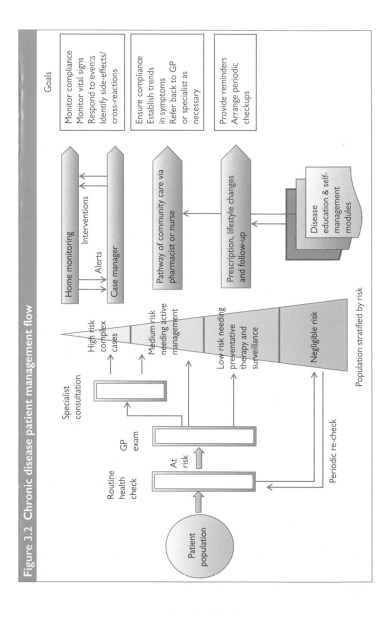

Diabetes, like all chronic diseases, is a process—leading step-by-step to decline if not managed well. Best practice care is also a step-by-step process, starting with prompt diagnosis—simple and inexpensive, but often not performed until symptoms appear.

Because these diseases take their course over years, even decades, it is not easy to manage them in a continuous way—along the so-called continuum of care. And several require the attention of multiple specialisms.

Commissioning the whole process, not the separate encounters or episodes of care, is the answer. The process should routinely screen people for risk and then assign them to the right process of management (see Figure 3.2).

Those lucky enough (or shall we say healthy enough) to have negligible risk can simply be asked to come back in a few years' time. Those shown to have a level of risk should be seen by primary care professionals and assigned to one of three categories:

- **Low risk**, requiring a preventative regimen of drugs, exercise or lifestyle change, with periodic check-ups to assess if symptoms appear or worsen

- **Medium risk**, needing active management by a care team or primary care clinic, perhaps following a pathway laid out by a specialist. Prompts to ensure compliance with the regimen would be sent to the patient's mobile phone, and 'disease education' modules on DVDs would help the patient follow his own progress. Periodic testing, often at a pharmacy, will be used to check for setbacks

- **High risk** or complex cases, which will be referred to a specialist and will require active engagement with a care team and nurse case manager. An in-home disease status monitor would send alerts to the case manager, who monitors the patient's situation, by home visits or by telephone, and anticipates developments before they require emergency admission to hospital.

The savings would be substantial: unscheduled admissions of patients with chronic disease represent the single greatest cost to the system.

Two US disease management networks are taking a 'process' approach to chronic disease. Optum Health (from United Healthcare) and Healthways, both funded by employers on a per capita fee basis, use nurse practitioners to make weekly calls to tailor and monitor chronic care. This also improves patient satisfaction. A recently reported study by the Johns Hopkins Bloomberg School of Public Health found that elderly patients with multiple conditions were twice as likely to regard their care highly if this kind of 'guided care' approach was used.

Even those not yet afflicted seriously with a chronic disease should pay attention to their 'health scores'. In the US, Ingenix, a provider of healthcare management software, assigns patients 'health scores' by examining drug prescription data. This is to help insurance companies to price their policies. But patients themselves should know their scores and work to steadily improve them.

Diabetes is a case in point. A major international study by physicians at Australia's George Institute followed over 11,000 patients with type 2 diabetes over five years. The result of better controlling blood glucose was a 10% reduction in serious diabetes complications, a one-fifth reduction in kidney disease and a one third reduction in cardiovascular risk. Process approaches to chronic care management do not just improve outcomes, they save substantial costs: the diabetes management programme in Asheville in the US has reduced the average cost of care by $2–3,000 per patient per year.

Grace, Jane's mother, was one of the first to receive an Alzheimer's Risk Profile, now just called an 'ARP'. Until the 2010s, Alzheimer's was diagnosed from the appearance of serious symptoms—memory loss, confusion, and so forth. And, of course, earlier detection was not particularly useful until real prospects of arresting or reversing the disease had appeared. Therapy designers also needed to deal with the fact that various different forms and courses of the disease had emerged from 'biomarker' studies on patient samples, showing different molecular signatures that foretold the different courses the disease could take. Each called for different therapies.

When drugs for these different forms of the disease had appeared, the ARP soon became standard practice for someone in their 50s and 60s. Grace's ARP test was a mixture of genetic and proteomic measurements. The genetics spelt out the probabilities and the protein tests showed the early steps leading to the formation of 'amyloid aggregates', which themselves were a step on the path to the tangles and plaques in the brain that marked full-blown Alzheimer's.

The first time the test was run on a sample of Grace's blood, it showed a high level of genetic risk but no early signs of disease. However, now that drug therapy was available, Alzheimer's had joined that list of chronic diseases that were managed carefully from the very beginning, and the doctor arranged for annual repeats of the test until the day when they showed that the molecular pathways en route to disease had begun to show themselves. At that point, Grace had no symptoms at all – she was still 'bright as a button'.

The disease management process that followed was centred on Grace as the patient, rather than designed for the convenience of the system. Gone were the days in which managing a chronic disease was a series of unconnected encounters with medical professionals, with the patient unengaged with the process and uninformed about it. After a discussion with the doctor, Grace was given an 'information prescription' laying out all that was known about the disease, the form it was likely to take, the schedule for further tests and brain scans and the medicines that would slow and with luck prevent the damaging changes to her brain.

She was assigned a nurse 'case manager' whose role was to check in regularly, ensure Grace understood the plan, had the chance to change it where necessary, and was following it: in other words, that it had become *her* plan. All the evidence was that chronic care plans that patients had helped create were also much more likely to be followed.

This 'process' approach requires some upfront investment, for routine screening and to establish the infrastructure to manage and support higher risk patients. But, if the result is that admissions to hospital are dramatically reduced, the long-term payback will be very positive.

Streamlining the development of new treatments

The cost of developing new technology is spiralling. Establishing benefit and risk and satisfying ever more risk-averse regulators, is becoming increasingly lengthy, complex, and expensive. Lengthier tests and more competitive markets mean that innovators have less time to recoup their investments. So prices mount even faster than costs. We are faced with a stark choice: either we simplify development and reduce its costs, or we forgo advance in medical technology.

Simply telling people they must accept less testing of new therapies and so more risk is politically unacceptable. We must 'work smarter, not harder' in establishing the benefit/risk ratio of new technology. This requires a fundamental rethink of the way in which we test new treatments, especially drugs.

We should start by questioning the mainstay of drug testing—the randomized controlled clinical trial. Introduced more than 50 years ago, it has become the gold standard of clinical evidence. Each trial is composed of two 'arms', two groups of patients selected randomly. One receives the new treatment, the other either the current treatment or 'placebo'. Neither the patient nor the doctor treating them knows which is which.

A series of trials, with increasing numbers of patients, moves from checking there are no major side effects, to finding the right dose to be used, to establishing that there is real improvement in outcomes, and finally to assessing this improvement versus the risks of rare side effects in a large group of patients. The final stage can involve tens of thousands of patients and take several years, and can be hugely costly. A recent single trial cost £180 million, or $300 million.

Each trial is analysed separately, with the knowledge acquired in the earlier stages discarded for the purpose of the next, in the search for statistical purity. Until analysis of each trial is complete the next cannot begin, resulting in 'dead time' in the overall process. And, as every schoolchild and shareholder knows, time is money.

The other major drawback lies in the selection of patients. In order to minimize accidental bias between the 'treatment' and 'control' arms, patients have to satisfy demanding screening criteria. The result is that the trial can be quite unrepresentative of the population that will receive the drug once approved for general use.

We need new approaches, some explored in an ancient British tradition—the Harverian Oration. The famous physician William Harvey, who discovered the circulation of the blood, left a bequest to hold an annual lecture and 'feast' at which a distinguished scientist could lay out new thinking. In the 2008 Oration, Sir Michael Rawlins, the former head of the UK Committee for the Safety of Medicines, dissected the current process and reviewed alternatives, including a 'learn and confirm' model now being pioneered in pharmaceutical development.

Instead of a sequence of artificial trials this model allows the new medicine to be used in a steadily increasing group of patients. So-called 'Bayesian' analysis is then used to decide if the results are adding up to an acceptable benefit/risk balance, or not.

Alternatively, 'case control' studies compare the results of a new treatment with those from past treatments on similar patients, avoiding holding back the latest treatment from the 'control arm' patients in the course of a trial.

In an article in the medical journal '*The Lancet*', I incorporated some of these ideas in a new and simpler approach to medicines development, resulting from discussions among senior regulators and medicines developers. It distinguishes more clearly different kinds of new medicines and applies seven new approaches to the problem:

- Forming innovative partnerships, between companies developing products, with academic groups, and also with health systems, to share costs and risks
- Streamlining the trials process, simplifying the over-bureaucratic 'Good Clinical Practice' guidelines and replacing many of the personal visits to clinical trial sites with electronic monitoring
- Co-designing the confirmatory trials between the innovator, the regulators, and the value assessment agencies, so that the trials are able to prove what each agency needs
- Defining acceptable benefit/risk ratios more scientifically, taking greater account of patients' views
- Applying new trial design and analysis approaches to build up a picture of benefit and risk over time
- Applying stratified/personalized medicine to the selection of patients, to reduce the patient numbers, and the time and costs for successful trials
- Collecting some of the information on a medicine's value to the system, and on rare side effects, *after* launch by allowing early 'conditional approval' for defined patient groups, making pricing more evidence-based.

The·new approach is illustrated in Figure 3.3:

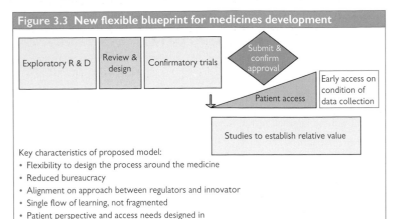

Figure 3.3 New flexible blueprint for medicines development

Exploratory R & D | Review & design | Confirmatory trials | Submit & confirm approval

Early access on condition of data collection

Patient access

Studies to establish relative value

Key characteristics of proposed model:
- Flexibility to design the process around the medicine
- Reduced bureaucracy
- Alignment on approach between regulators and innovator
- Single flow of learning, not fragmented
- Patient perspective and access needs designed in

The exact trial approach will vary from one technology, or drug to another: too much rigidity will continue the spiral of time and costs with no benefit to patients. The goal should be to halve the cost of development and so at least halve the cost of new technology.

Motor neuron disease, a slow but remorseless killer, brings great distress to the patient and all those near and dear to them. In some cases, like the famous physicist Stephen Hawking, some sort of life can be prolonged for decades, but only by the use of life support technologies.

When Jane's cousin **Robert** was diagnosed with MN in his 40s, it sounded like a death sentence—that is, until he heard about a new drug that, in early patient trials, showed real promise. The problem was that trials to fully demonstrate that the drug changed the course of the disease would take many years to complete—requiring a huge investment, difficult to justify commercially on the basis of the small size of the patient population. But it was clear to the discoverers and to the regulatory authorities, and of course to the patients, that—if the drug lived up to its early promise—it would be a tremendous breakthrough.

So all the so-called 'stakeholders' got together for a unique conference. The discovery company agreed to extend their trials in partnership with a number of health systems, who offered to conduct the trials free of charge. The patient organization agreed to connect willing MN sufferers with the trials, and Robert was one of the lucky ones. And the regulators agreed to

(Continued)

accept early biological markers of success rather than long-term recovery as the basis for widening treatment to others. As a result the trial was dramatically streamlined, and a much more cost-effective set of trials resulted in provisional approval for the drug within a couple of years.

Robert's disease was slowed, although not stopped, but the result was many more years of useful life. Without the agreement struck between the company, the patient organization and the regulatory authorities, the drug might never have seen the light of day. And Robert might never have gone on to head the International MN Society.

Intelligent targeting of care—the right medicine for the right patient

Too much health care is still 'hit or miss'. For example, it is estimated that on average 40% of medicines prescribed are unsuited to the specific patient who receives them, either because of inadequate efficacy or undesirable side-effects. With the medicines bill ranging between 10 and 20% of total healthcare costs, this is an enormous waste of resources.

With the genetic, proteomic and metabolic markers coming available, we can better target both 'blockbuster' therapies and more specialized treatments. New generations of medicines for common conditions like asthma, diabetes, coronary artery disease, etc. will be much more likely to justify prices that return their R&D investments, if they are efficiently targeted to those who do not respond well to current therapy. Highly priced drugs for cancer and immune disorders will require more precise targeting tests to establish value and secure adoption in tomorrow's health systems.

Personalized medicine is now gaining real momentum on both sides of the Atlantic. A Personalized Medicine Consortium has been created in the US and a new UK initiative is forming under the Technology Strategy Board and the Medical Research Council. Companies are springing up with genetic and proteomic markers, with algorithms to use test results to estimate risk of disease and benefits of therapy.

Discoveries made by such initiatives are, however, just the beginning. They need to be turned into routine, clinically validated tests, a process that will take several years and many millions. These must then be embedded in patient pathways, understood and adopted by doctors who today take a 'trial and error' approach. To ensure this happens, patients themselves will need to turn a natural concern that they are getting the right treatment into a personal interest in their personal care pathways. Such tailor-made pathways will command more patient adherence and hence get better outcomes.

To get the full benefit of genetic profiling to establish an individual's risks and responses to therapy, legislation must tackle two problems: employment risk and insurance blight. Congresswoman Louise Slaughter's Genetic Non-discrimination Act (GINA) prohibits the use of genetic information in deciding whether to employ or insure someone. Such provisions are needed worldwide.

Jane's mother-in-law **Rose** had for many years an occasionally painful and highly inconvenient bowel condition. Over that time, diagnosis had proceeded a long way from the crude irritable bowel syndrome (IBS) description she remembered from her first consultation with the doctor.

She had tried probiotic yoghurts, anti-spasmodic drugs, peppermint oil capsules, even hypnosis in case the problem was psychological, but nothing seemed to help for long. Recently much more precise biomarkers had been discovered that could pinpoint the biological mechanisms at work making the gut hypersensitive. 'IBS' had been sub-divided into eight different conditions with mechanisms varying from auto-immune disease to specific allergies.

It turned out that there was a particular bacterium in Rose's gut that induced the reaction and her unpleasant symptoms. Targeted antibiotic therapy eradicated it without any side-effects.

Life was suddenly simpler and much more enjoyable.

Making war on waste—waste not, want not

Waste in healthcare is a crime, one committed millions of times daily. One senior doctor in Britain estimated that one-third of health spending in the NHS is wasted. On the other side of the Atlantic, Dr Jack Wennberg of the Dartmouth Medical School recently made the same broad estimate. Peter Orszag, White House Budget Director, said in April 2009: 'Estimates suggest that as much as $700 billion a year in health care costs do not improve health outcomes. It occurs because we pay for *more* care rather than *better* care.' What an indictment!

Which one-third of healthcare, what $700 billion in US costs, are we talking about? Ineffective, unwanted and unproven procedures, replies Dr Wennberg. We could add to the list: drugs that are dispensed but never taken; surgical supplies ordered but thrown away; duplicated scans and tests.

CT scans are a notable example. Across the US, 62 million scans are conducted annually—one for every five people in the population. The scans are not only costly, they represent potentially harmful exposure to radiation.

No business would survive with this level of waste.

The challenge is identifying it. In some cases, it lies in specific procedures for which the evidence is poor or contrary to use. Examples are tonsillectomies, some prostate cancer surgeries (where 'watchful waiting' would be better) and many Caesarian sections (done for convenience not medical necessity). In these cases it ought to be sufficient to share the evidence with the doctors and patients, but several systems use incentives and penalties to discourage them.

In the UK, NICE recommends 'decommissioning' of services that are either outmoded or shown to be less effective than alternatives. The agency estimated £700 million worth of NHS savings from such actions—for example, reversible contraceptive devices in place of the Pill, which women often forget to take, resulting in unplanned and expensive pregnancies.

While the right medicine at the right time can be a very effective intervention in disease, too many medicines prescribed by too many doctors over too long a time can not only waste money but result in hospital admissions for side-effects or interactions. Sometimes over-medication becomes a spiral of decline, as different doctors seek to treat the symptoms of adverse drug reactions (from past prescriptions or 'alternative' herbal medicines) with yet more medication. Regular Medicines Use Reviews for older people, usually performed by the pharmacist, is the best way to tackle this problem.

Healthcare waste often lies not in what care is provided, but how care is delivered. For example: in-patient care, when community care would be an attractive alternative (such as much cancer drug infusion in Britain); surgeries that could be day cases that currently require hospital admissions; post-surgical stays that are longer than necessary.

Reducing these just requires better management. More challenging are questions of medical judgement—for example, the referrals that are done simply to rule out the improbable—where more experienced family doctors can reassure patients without a hospital visit and a specialist's fee.

Key to making such judgements more cost-effectively is minimizing defensive medicine, performed to reduce the risk of law suits. The first step is to reform the law so that lawyers do not have an incentive to press for extortionate settlements. The second is to provide for a defence that, by following clinical guidelines, a doctor was doing the best she or he could with the information available.

Much of the wasteful use of diagnostic and other precautionary steps would disappear, and the resources used where a real impact on care can be achieved.

The US system is mired in administrative complexity and cost. Striking estimates of administrative waste in the US came in a 2003 study advocating a switch to a single payer system, which claimed that the US wastes more on health care bureaucracy than it would cost to provide health care to all of the uninsured. Streamlining administrative overhead to Canadian levels would save approximately $286 billion in 2003, nearly $7,000 for each of the 41 million Americans who were then uninsured.

Empowering the patient—the best healthcare manager of all

A ground-breaking piece of work on the NHS was carried out for the British Government by Derek Wanless, who considered what would make the most long-term difference to the viability of the system. He concluded that it was engaging patients more actively in their own care. Only in the 'fully engaged' scenario, in which people took responsibility and action for improving their health could he see the prospect of a sustainable system.

People's willingness to engage and change has two dimensions – skill and will. *Skill* is a matter of giving people the right information and showing them how to act on it. In other words, giving people the 'power questions' they should ask their doctor and tuning the answers skillfully to their educational level and cultural background.

Will is a different and much tougher matter. Motivation is not created by mere information ('Smoking Kills'). It comes from within, as a result of a decision to either seek a positive outcome or avoid a negative one. Motivation varies with two factors: how pressing the problem is and how major the change needed. Immediate health problems—those that cause pain, or loss of critical function—act as their own motivators. If the change needed to improve health prospects is quite minor, like walking a little each day, or eating more fruit, then few outside incentives are needed. The real challenges are tough and sustained lifestyle changes that are needed to arrest the progress of a disease long before serious symptoms are felt.

One obvious way to develop the necessary will to change is to show people graphically what the future will hold if they fail to look after themselves. Better still, to show individuals two alternative outcomes of life courses, for example the two different paths a diabetic's life would take if the disease is well-controlled—or not.

It helps if it is an outcome that we can visualize personally. As an example all too close to home, my father had emphysema, a disease of the lungs. I saw him gasping for breath after the slightest exercise. So from an early age I was determined not to have similar problems. So I haven't smoked, and have sought the kinds of exercise, for example mountain treks, that develop or maintain lung capacity. I have no idea (having not had access to genetic testing for emphysema risk) whether I had a real risk, but this has not stopped me from acting to minimize it.

A second approach is to connect people to networks that encourage each other—slimming clubs and Alcoholics Anonymous are examples. Health plans should create incentives to join such networks, and to take the actions needed to stave off the progress of disease.

The third way to empower patients is to use financial incentives. While healthcare free at the point of need has been the founding principle of the

NHS, this ought not to rule out using financial incentives to overcome the 'will' problem. Requiring NHS patients to pay part of the cost of preventable conditions (or in the extreme refusing to pay for expensive 'rescue' operations like liver transplants if alcoholism has created the problem) frees up resources for those whose conditions cannot be prevented.

Charging modest payments for doctor visits, excepting of course the chronically sick or extremely poor, may make some people think twice before making appointments for minor conditions for which the local pharmacist has all the expertise and products needed. For these reasons, they are common in many parts of the world.

Medical savings accounts, where the majority of the spending is in the hands of the patient, can also empower the account holder to take the right action to safeguard his health. Catastrophic illness—cancer, heart attacks, etc.—would be exempt, but routine care, its necessity and its value, would be decided on by the patient, much as she decides on a meal, on a holiday, or on a new car.

Ideas like this will grate on many in Britain. Healthcare is different, they will say. This is an understandable reaction, but it springs from an old model of healthcare—welfare for the underprivileged—and a paternalistic mindset, viewing patients as unable to make right choices for their lives.

Positive incentives are probably the most acceptable, like life insurance whose premiums are linked to preventative action. Active membership of a health club, control of weight, tobacco, and alcohol intake, and regular physical exams and screening tests should all reduce the premiums, since they can all postpone the visit of the Grim Reaper. Premium reductions for 'good behaviour', in terms of regular health checks and exercise, should also be applied to private health insurance.

Susannah's father-in-law **Don** was over six foot tall, like his father. When he had his first full physical examination and life health planning session in his early 30s, the doctor took a complete history including close family ailments. In the course of this, Don recalled that his father had suffered a slipped disc in his 40s that gave him nearly a year of painful disability.

The doctor ordered an MRI of the spine, which showed very early signs of compression and wear on the lower vertebrae, perhaps as a result of his work in furniture removals as a young man. If this wear continued and he was to put his lower back under the wrong kind of asymmetric strain Don would join the legions of people with lower back problems and pain. She therefore prescribed Pilates for George to strengthen and sustain his core muscles. It also helped his balance and general poise and strength. And adherence to his exercise regime earned him positive points under his health plan.

There has been no sign of lower back problems, though Don is now in his early 60s. But he always remembers to lift with his legs and not his back!

Tailored top-up insurance plans will also have a role. With some drugs in areas such as cancer becoming too expensive for normal plan coverage, we will see insurance plans aimed specifically at these conditions, so that patients have access to the best available, even if this is not funded by the state or private plan in which they are enrolled.

Better self-care will be aided by networks of patients providing support and counselling for each other. Patient organizations are evolving from being largely volunteer-staffed and capable of only the most general support, to being professionally managed sources of real expertise. Some will be able to deliver better chronic care advice than a hard-pressed GP. When backed up by specialist web-sites like dLife.com (for diabetics) they can give the advice that patients need in their own homes directly from 'people like them'. Indeed, there is now a web site called PatientsLikeMe.com, which connects patients with others with a similar disease profile, enabling them to share experiences and advice.

Self-help approaches need to be funded, and many resource centres survive through commercial sponsorship (the videos on dLife have pharmaceutical trailers). However, properly accredited and responsibly managed e-resources have a huge part to play in transferring routine information and advice from the expensive setting of a hospital or surgery to the home desktop.

So, empowerment is not just a matter of telling people they must take responsibility. They need goals, and the information, tools, expertise, resources, and incentives to pursue them. It will also be hard for those in a poverty trap to make healthy living a priority. However, for most of us, personal goals and tools like these need to be integrated into our lives, or 'patient empowerment' will remain an empty slogan.

Valuing on outcomes—the true measure of performance

Everyone wants top quality in their healthcare. Payers want quality, but with productivity. But both quality and productivity have been assessed wrongly in the past.

'**Quality**' in healthcare has been assessed in terms of the reputation of the doctor, clinic or hospital. In the US, the regular US News & World Report tells us that Johns Hopkins, the Mayo Clinic and the Cleveland Clinic 'score big in six or more specialties'. To produce these rankings they look at reputation among board-certified specialists, death rates, quality of nursing staff and technology and patient safety. In the UK, particular institutions have strong reputations in specific disciplines, like the Royal Marsden hospital for cancer and the Brompton Hospital for heart and lung disease. In UK private medicine, the watchword for quality (and expense) is Harley Street, where many of the top specialists in all the medical disciplines practice.

'**Productivity**' for a health system has historically been measured by dividing the activity level (the number of hospital procedures, the number of beds occupied, the number of patients treated) by the cost. This naturally drives management to reduce costs while keeping up patient throughput. Not a recipe for maintaining quality.

Defined in this way, quality and productivity seem to be enemies of each other. This need not be so, as we see in many other walks of life. Both quality and productivity need to be redefined, with outcomes at the centre. For outcomes are the final arbiters of the quality of care and the effectiveness of a doctor, a clinic, or a health system. Some outcomes are immediately apparent—recovery from infection, for example. Some require patient reporting months later, as in pain or mobility after joint surgery. Others only emerge over years—fewer fractures because of better treatment of osteoporosis, for example.

Recently the renowned business school professor Michael Porter, an expert on competition in business, turned to examining the US health system. He saw plenty of competition, at many levels of the system, and asked why this had not created efficiency, as it would do in most industries. He concluded that the competition was 'on the wrong things, at the wrong time and in the wrong way'.

So he asked what was the right kind of competition and concluded that health providers and systems should be measured and compete on one metric alone—outcomes.

His second main finding was that achieving high quality outcomes was not an enemy of cost—it was its ally. Those hospitals and systems that scored best on outcomes also were among the lowest cost – because outcomes tend to improve with the sheer number of cases the doctor or the facility dealt with, and so did costs—following the so-called 'experience curve'.

Two kinds of outcomes matter to patients. Clinical outcomes are critical, in terms of cure rate, completeness of recovery, no recurrence of disease, quality of life after treatment. But the way patients feel treated by the system, how their fears or concerns are dealt with, and their follow-up care managed, count almost as much. 'Patient-reported outcomes' need to encompass both.

A recent study by a UK think-tank, the Office of Health Economics, investigated the feasibility of measuring outcomes for four very different conditions: elective surgery, mental health, COPD, and colorectal cancer. In most of these cases they found that rigorous, well-researched approaches to gathering patient-reported outcomes already exist. In addition to recommending routine collection of such measures as mobility (for joint surgery) or mood (for mental health) the study recommended that patients be asked about their experience: access to care, the quality of its coordination, the availability of choice, the system's respect for their dignity and confidentiality, the quality of communication and the support given to carers and family members.

Despite the obvious importance of outcomes, medical professionals often base their decisions on 'custom and practice' that has never been tested in the crucible of outcomes. Past examples include the prophylactic use of anti-arrhythmia drugs for patients after heart attacks (they actually increased the death rate) and the use of corticosteroids in acute brain trauma (they worsened the damage).

In contrast, the proper evaluation and communication of the positive outcome of a treatment can vastly improve care. For example, giving caffeine to premature babies to reduce their levels of sleep apnoea results in fewer cases of cerebral palsy. *1st Slide ?*

Medical practice should be based on evidence, scientifically collected and evaluated. Not, you would have thought, a complicated idea, but one that did not take hold until the 1980s, when the evidence-based medicine movement began.

If outcomes are the best measure of quality, how to assess value? For this, clinical evidence needs to be turned into economics, via health technology assessment (HTA). This task is approached differently across countries like Germany, France, Sweden, and the UK, but in these and many other systems it has become a central part of seeking value for money.

The concept of the 'QALY'—quality-adjusted life year—is quite widespread in assessing cost-effectiveness. It attempts to combine the impact of a treatment on health quality with the time over which the patient experiences the improvement. Despite its popularity among health economists, there are several major issues with the QALY. Are all periods in a person's life equally valuable? What to include in a measure of quality of life, and is it best judged by the sufferer or by the rest of society? Can we judge another's pain?

On this last question, research by Daniel Kahnemann, a Nobel prize-winning economist, shows that sufferers judge pain differently from how non-sufferers might imagine. If asked after a painful period how painful it was, the duration of the pain does not affect the answer. Only two things affect the answer—the greatest momentary pain experienced, and the level of pain at the end.

So the idea that society can achieve an objective measure of relative pain, or of relative life quality, is at best a hopeful approximation, at worst a delusion. HTA calculations should be used as a tool, not a rule—and clinical need, treatment innovativeness, and impact on the lives of the patient and their family should all be taken into account in judgments of value.

Paying for outcomes rather than just healthcare inputs, treatments or procedures, is also the best antidote to supplier-driven healthcare (treatments given because they are the domain of the specialist to which the patient is referred, who gets paid per treatment given).

Given the right information, patients will choose their specialist or treatment based on the outcomes achieved for previous patients. We trust the reports of other patients (especially friends and family) at least as much as the advice of professionals, who may have a vested interest. Seeing the outcomes from a range of patients with the same condition would be a lot more reliable than just asking someone we happen to know, whose precise condition may not have been the same as ours.

So collecting, analysing, and publishing outcomes must become central to creating a value-focused health system, to ensure both quality *and* productivity.

Moving care upstream—closer to the patient

We speak of the right patient receiving the right treatment at the right time. But we should add 'in the right setting', since the current pattern of where care is delivered is often far from logical or cost-effective. For both better patient service and convenience and for the greatest economy we need to move care as far 'upstream' as possible, from hospital wards to outpatient clinics, from hospital-based clinics to the community clinic, to the doctor's office or the local pharmacist, and ultimately to the home itself (see Figure 3.4).

Keeping people out of hospital is probably the single most powerful step we can take to manage healthcare costs. Hospital stays and treatment account for over half of the NHS budget, dwarfing the costs of primary care, of medicines and of community health services. Treating patients at home instead of in hospital saves an average of £450 a day in the UK.

While technology has evolved dramatically, the basic model of the general hospital seems frozen in time. It is designed to function as what Clay Christensen in his book '*The Innovator's Prescription*' calls a 'solution shop'— solving a wide variety of medical problems for a fee per case. It is run by department, rather than by patient-centred care process, and its doctors are trained to be individual practitioners rather than information-enabled team members.

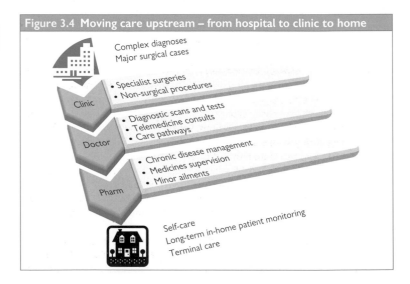

Figure 3.4 Moving care upstream – from hospital to clinic to home

Complex diagnoses
Major surgical cases

Clinic
- Specialist surgeries
- Non-surgical procedures

Doctor
- Diagnostic scans and tests
- Telemedicine consults
- Care pathways

Pharm
- Chronic disease management
- Medicines supervision
- Minor ailments

Self-care
Long-term in-home patient monitoring
Terminal care

For centuries, the general hospital has been seen as the emblem and focus of the health system. Opening a new one is a triumph; closing one is a disaster. Instead of viewing it as central, we should measure our success by our ability to keep patients from needing to cross its threshold.

The concept of the hospital, of course, originated in the days when little could be done for patients with major infections, terminal cancers or 'consumption' other than nurse them compassionately and hope that, if possible, nature and time might heal. As more and more could be done to intervene, it seemed natural to site the specialists and their new procedures in these same buildings, so that all patients could benefit from the existence of the range of facilities and know-how under the same roof.

The result—the modern tertiary care centre—is awesome in its complexity and cost. Patients with scores of different diseases follow labyrinthine pathways along corridors between specialists and departments, often returning to occupy beds while the specialists deliberate. As Christensen says, hospitals are 'among the most managerially intractable institutions'. High overheads and cross-subsidy between simple high volume cases and the more complex and costly ones, blur decision-making.

Many of the surgeries once performed in hospitals were by general surgeons for exploratory reasons. Now most surgeries follow quite precise diagnosis, with imaging and surgery being done in specialist surgical units, focused on knees, hearts, stomachs, etc. The costs and outcomes of these dedicated centres are frequently better than those achieved in the general hospital.

My own knee surgery, to deal with a torn meniscus, was carried out in a clinic by a doctor who carries out a series of such surgeries each session, with assistants and equipment designed for the task, with the necessary pre-surgical and recovery rooms needed to make it not even a day case but a half-day case. Nothing is gained, and there is more room for error and infection, when low risk, routine surgeries are performed in a general hospital environment. Of course, there are many unplanned surgeries—trauma cases, for example. But even here it is generally best to take such cases to dedicated, purpose-equipped and manned trauma centres rather than the local general hospital.

Turning surgeries into day cases rather than overnight stays is an obvious redesign step for more minor operations, yet there is huge variation in how far this is achieved. In just one small area of the UK (the East Midlands) the day case surgery rate varied from four out of five to one out of five!

The 'cost of complexity' of the general hospital can be crippling, but several hospitals have applied 'lean management' thinking to simplify flow and cut costs, much as engineering companies have streamlined their manufacturing. Improving patient flow and increasing direct care time for staff can improve productivity by more than 10%.

Some of the most advanced hospitals in the world, like the Cleveland Clinic, are breaking themselves up into a number of specialist institutes focused on neurology, or complex cardiovascular disease, where complex cases can

73

receive the attention of inter-disciplinary teams. Here the patients do not bounce between specialists in their various departments, but processes are designed to focus the necessary skills around the patient. This is the future for major tertiary care centres.

However, with the emergence of specialist elective surgery units, community-based diagnostic centres, telemedicine tools and online decision support, it is time to rethink the centrality of the 'big, white building'. There are several disciplines—dermatology for example—in which the specialist can just as easily perform both diagnosis and treatment in a community clinic as in the general hospital.

The greatest anomaly is the use of the hospital emergency department for minor ailments; a 'minor ailment' clinic in the high street or primary care centre is a much more cost-effective alternative. 'MinuteClinic' operates a network of such retail clinics across the US, offering treatment for 30 specific conditions, at a cost of between a third and a half of a doctor's office visit. They are situated inside high street pharmacies to minimize overhead costs, employing only medical technicians and nurses. They have experienced no malpractice suits, presumably because they set modest expectations within a strictly limited area of practice. And they free qualified family physicians for diagnosing, treating, and monitoring the more complex or less-easily recognized conditions.

With the NHS opening up to new models for private sector provision, experiments are beginning in the UK. 'The Practice' operates networks of GP practices alongside community clinics for ophthalmology and sexual health.

For the family doctor to remain an expert resource for the management of the more complex conditions, they will need three kinds of capability at their fingertips: on-line decision support, so that their diagnosis and treatment choices reflect the best clinical practice; access to community based diagnostics and imaging; and telemedicine links with specialists for the diagnosis and management of the most difficult cases. New diagnostics technology will be a big enabler of the shift of care upstream. In the past, the only way a physician could run a blood test was to send the sample to a nearby laboratory or hospital and wait two days or more to get the results. Now a chip is being developed that will measure the level of 35 proteins in 10 minutes. This could easily be sited in a primary care doctor's office.

This new role for the primary care doctor is far removed from the 'gatekeeper', standing in the way of access to specialist expertise. Instead he or she becomes a channel of that expertise, until a case comes along in which the doctor is genuinely 'out of his depth', or a patient has multiple conditions that defeat the decision support tools. Since a quarter of US retirees have five or more conditions, there is always going to be room for a community-based geriatrician who can manage their overall health.

The evolution of technology will assist the process of moving care upstream. Take heart disease. Not so long ago, the best approach to deal with heart attacks was to conduct open-chest 'heart bypass' surgery to sew a new artery in place. Then angioplasty came along – and a balloon was threaded through the bloodstream to expand the artery walls and enable the partially blocked artery to function again. For many patients that too has become unnecessary, as lipid-lowering drugs make the blockages fewer or less serious in the first place. The result is a move of 'demand' from the highest cost setting, the operating room of a tertiary hospital, to a 'cathlab' that can be based outside it, to the general practitioner's office or local pharmacist.

These developments will affect medical training. Currently all doctors pass through a period of intensive exposure to hospital medicine – so that they can deal with the most serious and complex cases, as well as deliver babies and treat minor infections. The best emerge as fine intuitive diagnosticians—able to spot the significant from a mass of detail and design the therapy based on what the seniors who trained them did in similar situations. It's still a craft rather than a science. As we move to information-empowered teams, the emphasis shifts from displaying individual flair and knowledge to the best use of information and the best leadership of teams. And perhaps, since an even larger proportion of doctors will be practicing in community clinics, more of the training should happen there.

Radical care redesign will not happen overnight, but can over a period of 20 years, given the right vision, information flows, and incentives. We must move as much care as possible out of hospitals to community clinics and primary care, and as much care as possible from these settings to the patient's home, with remote monitoring and skilled case management. Every admission to hospital should be seen as a failure of the ability to detect, anticipate, and intervene early enough.

A very special case for care in the home is our care for the terminally ill, especially the elderly. This is a point in life when compassion becomes more important than technology, which is chiefly useful as a means of creating comfort, not cure. Professor Keri Thomas, the UK's expert on end-of-life care, says that how we manage care for the terminally ill is the 'litmus test' of the effectiveness of a health system. A 'Gold Standards' framework enables professionals to design the pathway for each patient, and determine if care at home is feasible.

In the Netherlands the last year of life is estimated to account for 10% of total health costs, with three-quarters of this for hospital or nursing home care. A 1996 estimate for the total in the Unites States was 10–12%; for the state-financed Medicare system for retirees the proportion is much higher—about a quarter, with 40% of this in the last 30 days. About a third of these final month's costs can be saved by use of hospices and advance directives on treatment, avoiding heroic technology-based measures for extending life.

Assisting people to die at home with dignity and skilled support, if this is their choice, has real advantages for the patient and their family. Having observed this myself when my own mother died at home, it keeps the patient much more comfortable about their surroundings and gives the family unrestricted access at a time of great emotional importance.

The cost of end-of-life care for the over 85s is one-third lower than those dying between 65 and 75, an age range in which one would expect doctors and patients to expend more effort to extend life. The costs for those dying over the age of 100 are one-third less again. So, as populations age, the overall cost of terminal care may well decline.

But of course costs are not the dominant factor—the wishes and needs of the patient must be paramount. For the terminally ill, the clinical outcome is not the issue, but their experience is. Providing better support for those who wish to remain at home, laying out care plans that relatives and local nurses can follow, and applying intelligent compassion not just technology, will improve the patient's experience and the system's cost.

Jane's eye was caught by a yellowing photograph on the corner of her desk. Her grandmother, **Dorothy**—quite a beauty in her day. And she retained that beauty and liveliness into her late 80s. So it was a shock to the rest of the family, though perhaps not to her, when she received the news that cancer had taken hold. So she began a course of the new generation of anticancer drugs, to shrink the tumour and hold back its progress until her granddaughter's wedding, which she particularly wanted to see. On the day, she was one of the stars of the show, dancing with the groom, and the 'three generations' photograph showed how the family's bone structure had passed down from one beautiful woman to the next.

And Dot, as they affectionately called her, was still very much part of the picture when little Bernie came along, although rather thin and frail. At that point, the specialist counsellor from the local hospice laid out the longer term options for her and for the family. The first option was an attempt to remove the cancer by surgery. Even with the new techniques to minimize shock and blood loss to make the surgery safe for the elderly, the procedure had only a 30% chance of cure, and—since she was over 80—there would be a 70% co-payment, calculated on the basis of the failure rate for her age. Despite the cost, the family wanted her to consider this option. Next was a regularly rotated regimen of medicines, continuing her weekly visits to the community cancer centre. Although the people there were so friendly and efficient (she almost felt part of the family) the side-effects in terms of reduced energy and nausea were increasingly unattractive. The third option was managed decline – either at the hospice or at home.

She chose to die at home. Since still fiercely independent and still living alone, the first thing to discuss was supervision—she would need to wear a life signs monitor, agree to daily nurse visits and have her movements around the home eased by various devices to ensure she did not fall. Medicines for pain control, and ultimately intravenous feeding would keep her alert and attentive when the family came. And, in the final days, a new cocktail of medicines specifically designed to relieve anxiety without unwelcome sedation, made the process as bearable as possible for her and for the family.

(Continued)

Monitoring the life signs, and comparing them to millions of records of others, meant that the time of death could be quite accurately predicted. And so her parish priest and all the family were there. 'About as good a way to go as one could wish for', was what Jane said to herself as she smiled and replaced the picture.

So, clinical logic, patient experience and economics lead us to deliver non-urgent, minor, continuing, or terminal care outside the walls of the general hospital, in community clinics or the home. And to focus real emergency care in hospitals fully equipped for the task. Critically, we need a mindset change on the part of both the public and politicians who have regarded the hospital as an icon of healthcare, and a politically sensitive local asset to defend at all costs.

Aligning incentives—for more productive healthcare

Incentives work, even in the caring professions. To be more precise, incentives drive behaviour, for good or ill. Many of the problems of today's health systems are a result of incentives that encourage building excessive capacity, providing unnecessary treatments and holding on to patients who would be better treated elsewhere.

In the US, most physicians' income comes from the fees they receive from treatment. This is a powerful incentive to treat, and the risk of over-treatment results in tight pre-approval controls imposed by health plans.

This 'incentive to supply' is not restricted to the so-called 'private' health systems like the US; it happens just as powerfully in the UK's NHS. If hospitals are paid mainly in proportion to the number of patients they admit and the procedures they perform, they will tend to admit as many patients as possible and perform well-remunerated procedures on them.

To turn this around requires fundamentally new, productivity-focused incentive systems, for medical professionals, care commissioners and hospital management.

In the period 2000–2008, the UK poured new money into the NHS, largely in the form of higher pay for doctors and more medical and managerial posts. The total pay bill rose by over a third in just four years (from 2003 to 2007). The business case that won over the Treasury to the large pay increases was based on a steady year-on-year 1.5% improvement in productivity. Since, however, there was little real 'pay-for-performance' built in, the measured productivity actually declined.

The reason is not far to seek. In the UK, most medical staff are salaried; staff costs are over two-thirds of the total costs of the NHS hospital system. They receive automatic annual pay increments worth £420 million, with bonuses for good performance being relatively minor. Performance-related pay must become a much greater element of reward.

In contrast, among Britain's GPs, bonuses paid under the Quality and Outcomes Framework ('QOF') have indeed driven behaviour. Doctors have maximized the checks and treatments specified by the QOF, sometimes to extremes, putting people in their 90s on statins! Doctors also enthusiastically switched patients from one medicine to a less effective but cheaper one, under the influence of payments.

Neither family practitioners nor hospital specialists are rewarded for higher patient satisfaction, nor for better clinical outcomes. These should be the main factors that drive both financial reward and professional recognition.

Commissioners and systems managers also needed to be prodded in the right direction by appropriate incentives. One approach, favoured by the new Conservative-led government in the UK, is to put the bulk of commissioning in the hands of the GPs, the patient's point of entry to the NHS system. This would be a clear incentive to be frugal with both the therapeutic decisions they themselves take, and the referrals they make to specialists. On the basis of past experience (there was a brief period of 'GP fundholding' in the 1990s) this has a rapid impact on expenditure. Admissions to hospitals fell by 3% under 'fundholding'.

The challenges are equally obvious. If the person doing the commissioning also benefits from commissioning decisions, either by supplying the services themselves or retaining unspent funding, will their decisions always be in the interests of the patient? And can we expect GPs to have enough expertise to make sensible commissioning choices for rare or complex diseases, many requiring integrated care across several providers?

Getting incentives right for hospital managers is equally tricky. Fixing fees per procedure or case, via DRGs (the US system of 'Diagnostic-Related Groups') or PBR (the NHS system, 'Payment By Results') at least ensures that hospitals get paid in proportion to the numbers of patients they treat and the types of treatment delivered. But both systems represent an incentive to admit more patients and do more operations, so that fixed costs can be spread across more revenue. In fact a recent increase of 2.8% in PBR tariffs in the NHS resulted in overall hospital funding increasing by nearly three times that amount.

We need to reduce fixed DRG/PBR payments and reserve some part of the reward for achieving patient outcomes.

Incentives for patients can sometimes prevent the need for any treatment at all. Philadelphia scientists used a rigorous randomized controlled trial of smoking cessation to demonstrate that significant incentives ($100 for completing the programme, $250 for stopping smoking within six months and $400 for staying non-smokers) had a major impact on success. Those given the incentives were three times more likely to quit!

Alignment of incentives to keep healthy, screen for disease, manage chronic conditions well, intervene efficiently and achieve optimum outcomes can contribute powerfully to the productivity of the system.

Integrating care around the patient—using the power of information

Healthcare information is now coming out of the dark ages, from scattered paper records of isolated contacts between a patient and different medical practitioners, to a patient-centred record of a lifetime's journey through the system.

This will not only improve the delivery of care, it will save us a great deal of money: duplicated scans and blood tests; multiple clerical entry of the same information in scores of doctors' offices; side effects from the wrong medication; or treatment given but without positive effect, due to outcomes never having been properly tracked.

A fully functional information system will act as healthcare's nervous system, keeping track of what is happening to a patient (creating memory) and continuously analysing the value, or lack of it, from what is being done for this patient alongside results from millions of others (creating learning).

The patient's electronic medical record (EMR) will be central. So far it has been designed to meet the needs of either the doctor or the hospital: the one customer that has usually been forgotten is the patient. Future EMRs will carry the basic information from one care setting to another, and be available to the patient at home. No-one will be more concerned to ensure it is up-to-date and accurate than the person whose care it guides. However, there are still challenges to overcome—and ethical issues too: how much ability to allow patients to edit or hide the contents of a personal health record.

It is estimated that widespread adoption of interoperable personal health records could save the US health care system more than $19 billion annually *after* expenses. The use of this technology will spread slowly from health-focused or technology-literate enthusiasts to the rest of the population; it will be some time before we can make carrying them a requirement for using the health system, in the way that we ask drivers to keep their licences and insurance certificates in their cars. But that day will come.

As **Jane** glanced across her desk she saw her personal health card nestling in the home health card reader, supplied by her health plan. Although the reader was branded Excellent Health, her card could be read by any reader anywhere, once she entered the secure PIN code, just as it had been with ATM cards for decades. She recalled the number of times her health card had made a real difference to her healthcare. For example, when she was taken ill on holiday with a serious infection, and the card reminded her and, more importantly, the emergency room staff, that she was allergic to penicillin. Or when she was on a course of cardiac arhythmia pills that had to be taken on schedule each day, and the card reader reminded her with a sharp 'beep'.

(Continued)

(Continued)

She tapped the Excellent Health icon on her PC, and up popped the exercise regime that she and her primary care specialist had agreed, also loaded on the card. The card also fitted in the exercise machine in the corner of her bedroom: if she did the appointed walking and stair-stepping programme, the relevant number of plus-points would be added to her personal health account. The card also contained the care pathway—designed like a metro map—for the only ongoing course of care that she was currently receiving. The flashing 'station' on the care map showed the next step she needed to take: to place a finger-prick of blood in the biochip machine that simultaneously read over a hundred common blood test 'analytes', and then sent the result to her doctor and care manager.

All in all, she now could not now imagine life when all these simple steps in managing your own health relied on paper records, memory or needed a time-consuming visit to the doctor's office.

One of the benefits of seamless information is the power of comparison. While most doctors resent direction from others, they thrive on feedback that tells them how they compare with peers. Feedback on decisions made and costs incurred is used very effectively by the best US physician groups.

The same power exists with whole systems. One simple comparison of different regions across America is the cost per Medicare patient: it recently revealed that 10 leading regions averaged $1,500 less in costs per patient annually than the national average, while achieving better outcomes. The means used by each region to achieve quality and control costs was different—hospital consolidation in Asheville, elimination of unnecessary procedures in Cedar Rapids, and cross-community 'quality collaborations' in Portland. Imagine if each system could see not only what the others had done but the effects on quality and costs: the incentives built into the system should do the rest.

System-wide information on best practices is also the best way to resolve the tension between central direction and local entrepreneurism. As the Chief Executive of the NHS recently commented to me: 'We have to stop trying to solve the same problems 150 different ways!' (there are 150 different local systems in England).

New mobile technology and social media bring a plethora of new options for informing (or mis-informing) people. As more and more of our communications transfers to mobile devices, we can receive both advice and prompts—for example to take our medication.

The main value of integrated information is to open the door to integrated care, and this is a good note to end on in describing our 10 levers. In US experience, well-constructed **integrated health systems (IHS)**, like Kaiser Permanente and Intermountain Health, deliver consistency of care at affordable costs, and part of their secret is information flow. Connecting family doctors with hospital specialists, sending images automatically from radiologist to specialist to surgeon, and giving both clinicians and patient access to a complete health record—these are all more likely to happen and to influence care if all are part of the same organization.

In principle, the UK NHS should be able to operate as just such an integrated organization with a single information nervous system. This was the theory behind the 'Connecting for Health' programme, underway over the last five years. It has delivered some benefits, like the 'Choose and Book' ability for a patient in a GP's surgery to select where and when to see a specialist. However, it has been widely seen as an expensive white elephant and may not survive the next period of austerity in the NHS. But if we lose the ability to compile a comprehensive record and integrate care this would be a major lost opportunity to improve NHS performance.

Integrated health systems are hard to build and operate without installing bureaucracy and barriers to local innovation, but the full power of integrated information to design and deliver care around the patient is probably only possible within an IHS.

Using the levers—achieving the impact

Our 10 levers require courage to use, since they take everyone out of their comfort zone—patients, doctors, hospitals, and governments. The consequences will be radical change in where care is delivered, and in the roles of patients and professionals. We will need fewer hospitals, more investment in community diagnosis and treatment, more mobile professionals and greater use of modern information technology. But only such changes can make quality care affordable and sustainable.

Each lever alone makes a difference, but if pulled together they powerfully reinforce each other. Some examples include:

- Using evidence-based information to create best practice pathways will enable more care to take place outside specialized centres
- Putting the right incentives in place will encourage patient responsibility and engagement in prevention and self-care
- More targeted approaches to creating new medicines will streamline and speed their development, avoid waste, and enable more systematic processes of care
- Better chronic care processes, including remote patient monitoring, will assist in the design of lower cost delivery systems, with the deployment of the right level of expertise at each point, equipped with best practice information
- Tracking personal health signs via integrated patient-accessible health records and predictive tools will prompt the patient, with counselling from doctors or health coaches, to detect health warnings early and take preventive action

81

- The ability to capture and interpret the results of care across populations and through the lifetime of individuals will enable much more targeted or personalized care
- Empowered patients, equipped with portable health information, will play a much larger part in selecting providers or locations at which to receive their care
- Eliminating ineffective care given to individuals who will not benefit, or will suffer bad side-effects, will improve outcomes and reduce waste
- Rigorous analysis of outcomes through national benchmarking systems will propel the improvement of productivity
- Compassionate and cost-effective end of life care will be delivered at home by monitoring patients remotely, and supporting care givers with expert advice.

The greatest benefits come from pulling these levers together, and the best way of doing this is in an integrated health system.

The case for integration

Integrated Health Systems can achieve a number of things that are hard or impossible in today's largely fragmented health landscape. Firstly, by containing both primary and secondary care professionals and facilities they can optimize where care is delivered without a struggle for funds and for patient control between community- and hospital-based doctors. Secondly, they can take responsibility for the continuum of care for a population of patients, making chronic disease management more straightforward. This enables them to compete on patient outcomes and costs, and focus on the total patient experience, not on isolated encounters.

If their budgets are allocated on a per capita basis, and they have a long-term relationship with the population for which they are responsible, they have the incentive to invest in prevention and in the processes and technology for chronic disease management. This is in contrast to doctors, clinics, and hospitals whose contacts with patients are temporary and deal only with immediate health needs.

As technology evolves and best practice pathways change, an IHS can re-work how patients flow through the system, without the need to constantly renegotiate relationships between specialists and their primary care colleagues. Finally, they can build integrated information systems and mandate their use by all their professionals.

In other words, the ability of an IHS to integrate care around the patient, and to think and act for his long-term health needs, puts most of the 10 levers within reach.

How can we get there from here?

In the US, such systems have already proven their long-term appeal but aspects of health insurance still prevent their achieving their full potential.

Incentives for plan members to stay with a plan for a number of years, or to retain membership under similar terms when changing employers or retiring, would increase the incentive for the IHS to make long-term investments.

In the UK, incentives need to be put in place to encourage long-term relationships to be forged between the major academic health science centres, community clinics or hospitals, and primary care doctors, in order that the overall system can be commissioned on a population basis. Ultimately the IHS may own all the clinics and employ all the doctors but this is not necessary as a first step.

Where does competition come in? In major urban areas, like London or Los Angeles, there is room for a small number of competing systems. This competition for the loyalty of plan members and for their share of the health budget, will be on the basis of outcomes and costs. In rural areas, there may be room for only a single system, but incentives can to be designed for them to compete in performance with their peers caring for similar populations elsewhere in the country.

Whether within an IHS or by design of a system that pulls together independent units to act in a similar way, the goal must be to use the ten levers to transform the productivity of healthcare, while maintaining or improving its quality. We need to reverse the impact of the supply and demand drivers if we are to achieve sustainability (see Figure 3.5).

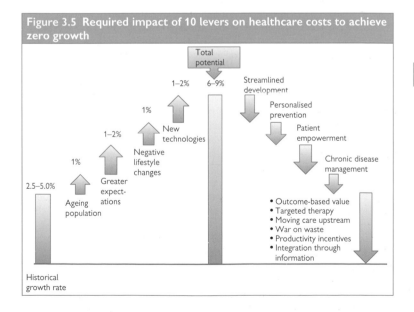

Figure 3.5 Required impact of 10 levers on healthcare costs to achieve zero growth

However, the best way to get a sense of how the 10 levers can combine to transform the quality and productivity of healthcare is to revisit Jane and her family doctor, Dr Clive Patterson, in 2030.

The 2030 Vision

Jane's care has become truly patient-centred. Genetic and other tests have given her and Dr Patterson a scientifically based sense for which conditions she is most at risk, and how she can improve the odds by her lifestyle. She knows which of the ailments her parents suffer are potentially in her future and what she needs to do about them, including annual screening tests and daily dietary supplements.

Her annual full body scan automatically signals when significant changes have occurred that might signal a potential tumour or other abnormality. And, depending on the amount of change and the probability from her profile, her doctor can order a blood test, a more detailed scan or simply 'watchful waiting' until the next annual check.

Her medication history, allergies and key aspects of her care plan are loaded on a smart card, updated with every visit to the doctor or pharmacist. And because she is enrolled in a personal health plan, she receives a monthly 'health score' that details the points she has earned from health-promoting activities, like her personal exercise plan, and compliance with her medication (since her 'smart' blister pack signals the taking of each pill).

So she has a personal health management plan to suit her unique biology and unique circumstances. With their permission, she can also see the relevant parts of her family's plans – especially important for her children and ageing parents.

The integrated information system connects her to her doctor for routine queries, weekly checks or requests for an appointment, and delivers all the relevant information to the Dr Patterson's desktop. If she gets a diagnosis of a disease – acute or chronic – she can quickly access the sources of medical expertise most relevant to the disease, including patient-level 'health briefings' by well-known video doctors. She can also connect to other patients and learn how their disease was treated, what they felt about the process, and the steps they took to get the best outcome. When she receives treatment herself, the system prompts her to report key outcome measures, adding to the system's database.

With most common conditions now treatable rather than potentially fatal, she has lost the fear of the unknown that kept previous generations from consulting the doctor, and lost the feeling of helplessness in the face of a diagnosis. Put simply, she is in control.

(Continued)

84

The changes to **Dr Patterson's** life are no less profound. As he enters his office and voice-activates his information system, he automatically receives all he needs for an effective day in the clinic. First, the list of key medical markers for the patients he is actively manageing, with their overnight readings, compared with recent trends. The care pathways that are displayed help him decide if intervention is needed and if he needs to call the patient in. Second, he sees his e-mails, neatly arranged in three folders: patient queries, responses from other medical professionals on his patient care teams, and biomedical research updates on those diseases in which he specialises.

When he has dealt with these, he sees his first patient of the day. His health card updates Dr Patterson's system with health events or care received since his last visit. His symptoms suggest a severe respiratory infection, so he asks him to walk along to the clinic's diagnostic laboratory to identify the gram-negative bacterium that is causing the trouble. Based on the result, the system recommends the most effective antibiotic and the care pathway that the patient should follow, including an automatic chest X-ray in seven days if the symptoms of pneumonia should appear.

His second patient shows him the sore knee that resulted from a fall, and the flag on that patient's chip directs Dr Patterson to the recent MRI scan. It shows a meniscal tear that could easily have worsened to the point of needing surgery and so he shows the patient a list of potential knee specialists to consult, with the locations, costs and outcomes achieved. He also gives the patient access to health education software with an 'information prescription' containing images of the problem, the treatment and the potential effects of anti-inflammatory medication and physiotherapy.

Patient number three is a long-term Type 2 diabetic fitted with with an artificial pancreas, combining pancreatic stem cells with a smart biocompatible device that gives a read-out of the insulin, glucose and HbA1C readings for the last month. The decision support system indicates that the implant may need replacement.

Patient four has begun to suffer from palpitations and needs an ECG. The apparatus analyses abnormalities automatically and connects to a database at the regional cardiology centre. Comparison with the traces from other patients highlights a high probability of a cardiac event in the next few months and recommends an immediate referral. In parallel Dr Patterson orders the proteomic profile that he knows the specialist will need to check for atherosclerosis.

Intelligent anticipation, personalized medicine, and speedy, cost-effective response to problems: this is Healthcare 2030, if we use our levers to full effect.

Chapter 4

Taking responsibility—a healthcare agenda for the next 20 years

Healthcare is without doubt a hot issue, politically and personally. In a 2009 survey of young (30 years old or less) Americans, 96% agreed that that 'the healthcare system is broken and needs fundamental change'. 93% of them attributed this, at least in part, to 'an epidemic of chronic, preventable diseases'. It's not surprising. At current rates of increase, by 2060 when this rising generation are elderly, the whole US government budget will be consumed by healthcare! So even those who have little need for the system today worry that a wave of health system failures and costs will threaten to submerge their generation in future years. The rising generation also senses that healthcare technology will open up yet more exciting possibilities to improve the quality and quantity of their lives. But they also realize that healthcare systems struggle to fund today's needs, let alone the rising expectations of their ageing parents' generation that will drive up demand for health services at an ever-faster pace. Together these forces drive pessimism about the future.

We have seen how determined action with 10 powerful healthcare levers can reconcile these supply and demand forces and avoid the catastrophe of unaffordable healthcare. However, we also know how quickly politics and vested interests hamper necessary action on the health agenda. It is up to all—governments and healthcare system managers, medical professionals, and all of us as patients—to take responsibility if we are to have a high quality yet affordable future health system. The action agenda begins now.

While some of the 10 levers of change can take effect quickly—cutting out waste, for example—most of them have their full effect only over a period of several years. Prevention and better management of chronic disease, enabled by integrated information and the empowerment of patients, will reap huge returns, but over decades. We will often have to invest more in the short term to reap these future returns. Better targeting the care we deliver, moving it upstream towards the community and the home—these also require upfront investment so that our future healthcare achieves better outcomes for lower costs. And streamlining technology development so that future innovation is more affordable will only begin to pay real dividends in terms of lower costs and prices from 2020 onwards.

This long-term nature of the payback makes action now even more important, since delay will leave us with the only alternative: radical cuts and crude rationing policies. But where does the responsibility for pulling each of the levers lie?

Governments cannot escape a central role, shaping the landscape for the action of all the other players in the drama. They should ensure comprehensive coverage is available and structure the system so that payers and providers can compete effectively, with real patient choice, made on the basis of guaranteed minimum care standards and reliable outcome data. Governments must also monitor overall spending and control the health budgets that they raise and spend, while recognizing the link between better health and economic prosperity.

Employers can go further, encouraging the right kinds of screening, early intervention and health maintenance programmes. They need to exercise 'enlightened self-interest' to maximize the health and productivity of their employees. Their role is particularly important in the US where they are likely to remain major funders of healthcare for the foreseeable future.

Health system managers and commissioners of care have some of the most powerful levers. The ways in which they commission care can encourage good end-to-end health management and cost-effective delivery. They can mandate joined-up IT systems to manage care pathways, integrate care around the patient, and report outcomes consistently. They can also anticipate and incorporate new treatment options into these pathways and encourage the steady elimination of old technology and practices that no longer add value.

Health professionals deliver most of what we care about in healthcare and remain the most trusted parts of the system. They will still have a critical part to play, even in an era of standardized pathways and shifts of care to lower cost, more convenient settings. Primary care practitioners' skill in detecting and managing chronic disease will be central, as will specialists' ability to use best practice technology matched to patient need. Both will need more effective and frequent in-service training if they are to keep current over their careers, as streamlined technology development delivers change ever more rapidly.

But the greatest change must be in how all of us—**as patients, families, and communities**—take responsibility for our own healthcare. New tools and incentives, from personal risk assessment to portable health records, will focus, prompt, and encourage us to make management of our own health a greater part of our lives. For without our own more disciplined efforts, self-inflicted conditions will continue to rise, other diseases will be caught too late for the best treatment and all the other changes to the healthcare system will be for nought.

A health manifesto for governments

Healthcare is an inescapable issue for governments, right, left, and centre, across the world. Tackling it requires all governments to lift their eyes from today's emergency, urgent budget priority, hot media issue, to shape the landscape for sustainable healthcare. Some may say that governments never act long term: they are always dominated by today's news headlines, by what the latest opinion poll says will get them re-elected. But, if this were always true, countries would not have road or railway networks, effective defence forces, or nuclear physics facilities. Where governments perceive a long-term strategic priority and can explain it to voters, they invest for the long term. There is no more critical strategic priority than the health of the population.

In 2007 the number of over 65s in Britain overtook the population of working age for the first time, so that those paying into social insurance schemes become outnumbered by those most likely to draw on them. In the US, there are dire predictions of the bankruptcy of the Medicare system that takes care of the retired. Action to balance the health care budget is a pressing political issue on both sides of the Atlantic. Of course, the political debate on the two sides of the Atlantic comes from opposite directions. In the US the main concern is that government involvement will erode individual rights to access the best care. In Britain the issue is whether government-funded healthcare, under new budget constraints, can deliver all that people need. However, the government is a major player in both cases, funding 90% of British healthcare and more than half of the US bill.

However, *governments should only do what only they can do*. They are not good at new technology development, at fixing the right price for health technology, and at ensuring that best practice medicine is actually practised. But they cannot stand back from responsibility for creating the right conditions for sustainable healthcare. First, though, they need to realize that investment in health also makes sound economic sense.

Shifting political thinking, from health spending as a burden, to an investment

Spending on healthcare has long been considered a burden on the economy— either directly a cost to the public purse, for a government-funded system like the UK's, or as an indirect tax on an employer, in the form of employees' private insurance coverage, as in the US. This outlook is understandable, since healthcare jostles for funding with other critical public priorities, like education or defence. Or, equally, when General Motors has to pay more in health insurance than it does for steel, it helps drive the company into bankruptcy. Understandable as it is, this 'healthcare as burden' mindset is wrong. Economically intelligent healthcare can improve the productivity of General Motors' workforce. A productive healthcare system is a key national economic asset. Countries without effective health systems will suffer a disproportionate burden of disease, resulting in workforce absenteeism or under-par performance, and will not be able to keep large numbers of people in their 60s and beyond in productive employment. They will slip down the league table of global competitiveness as nations, because they are either not spending enough on health, or not spending it in the right way. The US is more vulnerable than most. Now spending more than any other nation—16% of its GDP—on healthcare, it is far from getting value for money. On most of the simple, basic measures of quality, it lags behind countries with much lower levels of spending. It has a shorter life expectancy and a third more healthcare-preventable deaths than most other developed countries and its infant mortality rate is seven per 1,000 births, compared with an average of 2.7 elsewhere.

Yet, as we have seen in the fierce opposition to the Obama health plan, the US is deeply attached to the status quo and to its vested interests.

There is, of course, also a strong positive link between prosperity (GDP per head) and the share of national wealth spent on healthcare. But does healthcare expenditure boost prosperity and stimulate economic growth, or simply allow countries to channel more resources into 'feel-good' activities that add little to their economies? The answer is: it depends! Some health care is economically intelligent, some is socially justified, and some is neither economically nor socially compelling. See Figure 4.1.

Economically productive healthcare does not just make patients feel better, it improves the personal productivity of the patient, carer, or family member as employees or homemakers. Often a positive outcome will return someone to the workforce, or allow them to work at full effectiveness for longer and retire later. The increase in personal 'lifetime productivity' offered by better health outcomes is of growing importance as the ratio of those in

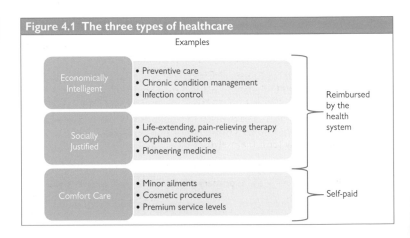

Figure 4.1 The three types of healthcare

Examples

Economically Intelligent
- Preventive care
- Chronic condition management
- Infection control

Socially Justified
- Life-extending, pain-relieving therapy
- Orphan conditions
- Pioneering medicine

Reimbursed by the health system

Comfort Care
- Minor ailments
- Cosmetic procedures
- Premium service levels

Self-paid

work to the total population falls. To compensate for this we need the lifetime productivity of current workers to increase by at least 10% every decade. Otherwise tax-funded health budgets (or those available from corporate profits) cannot keep pace with society's healthcare needs.

Early diagnosis or intervention in chronic disease are some of the most economically productive investments a health system can make, yet all too often are budget casualties in times of short-term economic pressure. Likewise, vaccination, screening and monitoring to prevent, delay or detect otherwise costly or catastrophic conditions are economically intelligent. Others are insurance policies for the future: pandemic vaccines, anti-viral treatments, and stock-piling of strategically important medications are strategic investments to avoid the collapse of health systems or economies if the worst happened.

The second category of 'socially justified' *healthcare* is the most problematic for policymakers. Treatments to extend the life of terminal cancer patients, or to save the lives of brain-damaged children or accident victims, fall within this category These kinds of health expenses can only be justified by society's compassion, tempered by judgment about whether the outcomes achieved for the costs incurred represent a better use of resources than other 'socially justified' needs.

Also in this category, in my view, come pioneering treatments (such as new organ transplants, novel cancer drugs, and experimental procedures). Without these innovations, no real advance is possible, and society is the loser in the long term. Factoring into the policy equation the impact of such inventions and their commercialization on economic growth should persuade policymakers in countries with vibrant life sciences sectors to broaden what they support. It is not logical (at least to me) to measure spend on these kinds of treatments against economically justified care: end-of-life cancer care should not be compared with prevention of diabetes. It is only the policy assumption that the healthcare pot is fixed, irrespective of what it is spent on and its long-term impact on the economy, that drives this kind of comparison, beloved of the current UK system.

We need to find a long-term funding formula for 'economically intelligent' care that reflects its wider impact on the economy, and use our combined clinical and economics skills to design the most effective use of resources to reduce the disease burden. For 'socially justified' care we should consider central funding, allocated to types of treatment or individual cases by panels of citizens, ethicists and clinicians, supported by health economists. Our third category, 'comfort care', should be easiest to manage politically—by eliminating it from national system or health plan coverage, while of course allowing people to pay for it themselves.

Rethinking public health—as personal and community health

Public health—long seen as a primary responsibility of governments—has some major triumphs under its belt. Sewer systems, clean water supplies, childhood vaccination, and the banning of smoking in public places have all had massive impact on general health and life expectancy. But we have also learned its limitations. Despite huge publicity campaigns, the wish to smoke, drink or eat to excess, and to take a myriad of other health risks is, so to speak, alive and well.

Information and education that reminds us of what we already know, and exhorts us to do the unpalatable, has little impact on the choices we make. We cross our fingers and hope we can escape the consequences. However, we are moving into the era of predictive medicine, in which we will know the diseases to which each individual is most vulnerable, and the behaviours they should avoid. It is time to rethink 'public health' and turn it into community and personal health maintenance. Personal health will profile individual risks, deliver personalized messages, and monitor health status, reinforcing individual responsibility for our health future.

Much of the investment in this new era of personal health should come from health plans and providers, but governments need to lay the groundwork by investing in the research needed and legislating for health coverage that includes personal prevention plans.

Accelerating personalized medicine

The science to better target therapy is progressing in leaps and bounds, but turning it into practical tools for routine clinical use is not. The way our R&D efforts are structured is unsuited to the task. Academic researchers are uncovering a myriad of possible markers, but lack the experience to distinguish the practical from the impractical. Some of these discoveries are taken forward by 'biomarker' companies, funded by venture capitalists, but these typically lack the resources to properly validate them.

Meanwhile, the pharmaceutical companies, whose products need the biomarkers to target them, lack not the money but the expertise. Although many proclaim that no new drug candidate is allowed to go forward without an accompanying biomarker, they have little experience in selecting the most practical markers, or developing them into commercial tests. Some have the unrealistic expectation that major diagnostics companies will invest to bring these new targeting tests to market. They forget that these companies operate on much thinner profit margins and do not have the track record of doing the early stage clinical validation work. They prefer to market the tests once they have established themselves in widespread clinical practice.

So personalized medicine risks becoming becalmed in a kind of Bermuda Triangle, between biomarker innovators, pharmaceutical developers and diagnostic companies.

This is an unusual opportunity for constructive government intervention. They should back consortia of academics, 'biomarker' companies, and major pharmaceutical and diagnostic manufacturers and research charities to target diseases demanding more personalized therapies.

The US government issues 'grand challenges' to researchers to develop leading edge technologies for markets that do not yet exist. Remote-controlled surgery, artificial retinas for damaged eyes, and fast tests for infectious diseases have all emerged from such funding. On a smaller scale the UK government supports initiatives like informatics for clinical research and Stem Cells for Safer Medicines, and is considering a national technology platform for personalized medicine. So the race is on for leadership in the new world of convergent health technology. Governments must also tackle the regulatory challenge: the regulation of medicines and diagnostics are completely different processes. Combination ('combo') therapeutics and diagnostics will need new regulatory approaches, and these should quickly become global, to speed their arrival.

So, if governments want better targeted therapies they will need to take action to shape the markets and regulations to make this possible.

Tackling medical liability law

At least 10% of US health costs are driven by defensive medicine. As other cultures become more litigious, medical costs elsewhere will rise. Governments have a clear need to act, either to limit damages or define more narrowly what constitutes liability. Strict limits to punitive damage awards would appeal to doctors and hospital administrators, and rather less to patients and their lawyers. Of course we need to deal with cases of flagrant negligence that call out for justice. But increasingly, as we use our information systems to guide practice and analyse outcomes, we will be able to exempt doctors and their institutions from liability claims if they have followed best practice pathways that avoid unnecessary tests or procedures.

Shaping the health insurance landscape

Most importantly, governments create the conditions under which the rest of the healthcare sector operates, especially the structure of health insurance, whether publicly or privately funded.

Virtually all countries have a mixture of public and private health insurance. The key question is not the exact proportions of public versus private insurance versus self-payment, but how each is structured, and what it is allowed to cover and to exclude. Public insurance (either via general or health-specific taxation) or mandatory private insurance are needed for the major, unpredictable health events that can bankrupt an individual. Likewise, self-payment is logical for simple treatment costs for minor ailments via over-the-counter medicines, and most forms of cosmetic surgery.

The controversial issues are the costs of chronic disease (especially when preventable), of regular physical exams and screening procedures, and of elective surgery. How far should these be state-funded and how far privately funded? The new factor here is our growing ability to predict and prevent the emergence of diseases, and to arrest their development, by how we live. Health plans must incentivize patients and medical professionals to take the necessary steps to detect and prevent disease, by funding screening tests. They should also be prohibited from excluding or penalizing patients on the basis of the results. Secondly, we need to reward patients who make the necessary changes in their lifestyles, for example by excluding them from co-payments that would otherwise be required.

So, governments must act to shape insurance systems around the right basic principles—universal coverage, a focus on economically or socially justified care, evidence-based medicine, and providing incentives for long-term investment in better health, on the part of both plans and patients.

Governments can also publish basic principles to guide the system's development. The UK government recently published an 'NHS Constitution', to enshrine patient rights and responsibilities. The Australian government has articulated healthcare 'design principles', such as being people- and family-centred, and promoting equity, shared responsibility and wellness. These sit alongside 'governance principles': taking the long-term view, ensuring transparency and accountability, and encouraging a public voice and community engagement.

Of course the form that government action takes will reflect national culture and political attitudes. Right wing thinkers will prefer more private finance and a greater mix of market mechanisms, and a left wing policymaker will seek to raise more of the funding via tax and structure the system from the centre. The key thing is not the amount of market-making or central structuring. The key thing is whether the system they define can use the 10 levers effectively. Most of these levers are in the hands of others, and wise governments realize this (see Figure 4.2).

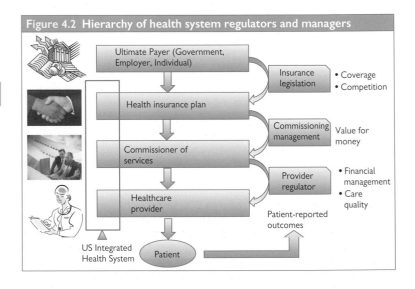

Figure 4.2 Hierarchy of health system regulators and managers

A challenge to employers

Employers have a long-term interest in the health of their employees, since they are typically the firms' most important assets, whose productivity can vary enormously with their state of health.

Health checks at work are therefore now quite commonplace in the US and in many European companies. Third party companies are used, to avoid employee concerns about confidentiality, and offer blood pressure, glucose, and cholesterol tests as well as obesity and lung function assessments.

For example, dedicated mobile health screening units now tour the stores of Lowe's, a national US retailer. The emphasis on voluntary personal engagement in the programme is an important feature, as the HR head says: 'When employees choose to take a health risk assessment and participate in the health screening, they become actively engaged in their health and are able to get personal advice for their health needs. Over time, we will have a healthier, more productive work force'. Another employer in the US, Lincoln Industries, has seen a huge drop in healthcare costs ($2 million a year) since initiating a wellness programme, with 'worker's compensation' claims, for healthcare costs from accidents, falling almost to nothing.

A major UK electrical utility company is going further, offering its employees the 'polypill', a daily dose of drugs to lower blood pressure and reduce heart attacks and strokes, prescribed by company doctors to those over 55, after a health assessment. It has stirred predictable controversy: one Member of Parliament said 'Companies do not have any business encouraging employees to take medication in their private lives'. But why draw a distinction between health screening and health maintenance?

Employer action is particularly important in the US, where employees switch health plans frequently, reducing the plans' incentives to invest in screening and early intervention.

A new focus for healthcare system managers

In contrast to governments, which should stick to creating the right regulatory and legal framework and the ground-rules for insurance plans, the leaders and managers of the health system itself must use as many of the 10 levers as possible, to drive productive change.

Creating effective competition—in commissioning and provision

Competition creates energy and spurs excellence. But not all forms of competition support the levers for change: for example, health plans competing for the least sick patients, or hospitals competing to build shiny new facilities to expand their capacity. In contrast to the US, where competition is endemic, in Britain it has been a foreign concept for most of the life of the National Health Service. Only in the last 20 years has a measure of real competition emerged, although so far only in provision, not in commissioning. The healthiest form of competition is in quality of care and outcomes for patients. League tables for surgeons or hospitals showing the outcome from operations, or the quality of chronic disease control in the case of primary care networks, will drive the right choices from commissioners of care and from patients.

Commissioning—for outcomes and value

Commissioning healthcare is rather unique, arising from the fact that the patient typically has neither the skills nor the control of resources to define and purchase the services they need. Someone else—the commissioner—acts on their behalf to define the service needs for particular groups of patients, and what the successful provider will be paid. To quote the NHS definition of commissioning: 'The process by which the health needs of the population are defined, priorities determined and appropriate health services purchased, evaluated and put in place'.

The way in which care is commissioned from providers has profound effects. Historically, most commissioning was focused on the interventions and procedures to deal with late stage disease. Primary care physicians were rewarded for consultations and hospitals were rewarded for their ability to admit patients for operations. So there was little incentive to prioritize prevention or take an end-to-end disease management approach.

'Capitation' in the US, offered by 'Health Maintenance Organizations' (HMOs) had the potential to deal with the problem. Insurers would only pay a certain amount per patient for total care and it was up to the healthcare providers to bid for the business of managing a total population. There was one immediate consequence—providers discovered that they did not understand their costs and so made wildly inaccurate bids. However, even after better costing was in place, the plans proved unpopular with patients, since plans balanced their budgets by restricting choice and limiting treatments.

In Britain, the budgets given to the local health boards are effectively capitated, but many aspects of commissioning are centrally controlled via fixed tariffs. Commissioners (currently the Primary Care Trusts, the PCTs) have a monopoly, resulting in a rather unequal struggle with providers. This system seems no more effective than the US at ensuring the right balance between prevention and treatment, and at adopting the best approaches to chronic disease management, to keep patients out of expensive hospital care.

Effective commissioning is the pivot-point of an effective health system. Only if commissioners are incentivized to think and plan long-term, will the right driving forces be in place for several of the levers: personal prevention, chronic disease management, personalized medicine, and care redesign, for example.

Payment systems have a key role to play. Currently there is a strong incentive for general hospitals, needing to support large overheads, to hold on to high-volume routine procedures that are much better carried out in dedicated facilities. The system needs to incentivise tertiary care centres to focus instead on the complex diagnostic challenges and high-risk patients and procedures for which they are best suited. Similarly, primary care providers need to be rewarded for their effectiveness in end-to-end management of disease populations, with performance measured by outcomes, not activity.

In the US, competitive commissioning, by health plans vying for the business of payer and patient alike, is a familiar feature of the scene. However this competition is still largely on the basis of premiums charged and freedom of access to providers, rather than outcomes. And frequent switching between plans hampers long-term prevention measures.

In the UK, competitive commissioning is overdue. If citizens could choose who is best placed to commission their care, based on relationships with providers and outcomes achieved, this would put commissioners on their mettle as never before.

Embracing care redesign

Health system managers need to be more open-minded than ever before, if we are to drive care upstream. With consumers and patients living different lives, the roles of doctors, nurses and pharmacists changing and new technologies for diagnosing, treating, and communicating available, new healthcare system designs are essential. Accordingly, experiments are springing up across the US (Mayo's SPARCS model and Kaiser's Garfield Centre) where the 'living laboratory' approach enables health managers to experiment in delivering new models of care.

These are very different to the incremental changes managers usually make. They are attempts to 'design from scratch' care delivery systems to meet current patient needs, to make full use of technology and to take full advantage of the skills of the coming generation of clinicians.

System change also has to be information-led. Catholic Healthcare West operates a chain of hospitals across California, Nevada, and Arizona. They recognize that in some of their locations they simply provide episodic care—taking care of someone facing one disease episode or injury. In others they offer 'continuum of care management' by working with groups of physicians. Their ultimate goal, achieved in parts of their network, is to offer population management, including the health plan itself.

One of their secrets to their improved performance is measurement—data, data, data. They collect and compare huge amounts of information on care quality, patient satisfaction, and financial performance systematically across their system, and use financial tools, bonuses, peer-to-peer competition, and plain top-down management authority to drive improvement. But such information transparency does not come cheap: they are spending $1 billion on IT systems over a seven-year period.

Managing providers—aligning methods, mechanisms, and metrics

If commissioners increasingly pay for performance, in terms of outcomes achieved on disease populations, the pressure will be on providers to manage their operations to this standard. What are the management tools at their disposal? The '7S' model we used when I was a consultant with McKinsey lists seven key methods and mechanisms available (see Figure 4.3).

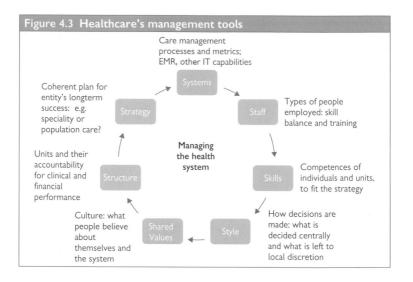

Figure 4.3 Healthcare's management tools

Care management processes and metrics; EMR, other IT capabilities

Systems

Coherent plan for entity's longterm success: e.g. speciality or population care?

Strategy

Staff

Types of people employed: skill balance and training

Managing the health system

Units and their accountability for clinical and financial performance

Structure

Skills

Competences of individuals and units, to fit the strategy

Culture: what people believe about themselves and the system

Shared Values

Style

How decisions are made: what is decided centrally and what is left to local discretion

For an effective healthcare system, all of these need to be aligned. This is rarely the case.

Central decision-makers like to focus overly on *structure*: shall we have 10 regions, 15 regions or abolish the regional level entirely? Structure change—particularly politically driven—rarely leads to a change of effectiveness of the system.

It is usually the performance management *system*, including measures and incentives, that has the greatest impact, for good or ill. For example, in the UK, NHS managers are measured by adherence to rigid annual budgets whilst senior clinicians are rewarded for clinical excellence by a jury of their peers. This is a recipe for the two groups pulling in opposite directions. Both need to share service line targets, in terms of quality and cost.

Management *style* is also critical. In the UK there is a lively debate about the right management style for the NHS. In the last few years we have seen very specific targets set from the centre—for example for the time to make GP appointments or specialist referrals, and time-to-treatment in emergency rooms. These have had a major impact on measured waiting times but have also had unintended negative consequences. Some have been 'gaming the system': ambulances 'going around the block' to avoid patients entering hospital before they can be treated is hardly a contribution to real performance!

An alternative to central targets is publishing outcomes, in terms of clinical results and patient experience, and then leaving peer pressure (and patient choice) to drive improvement.

Getting the *staff* mix (between qualified physicians, nurses, ancillary staff, and pharmacists) right is key to ensuring the best care for the fewest resources. A few talented clinical leaders will be more effective in leading performance improvement than multiple layers of non-clinical management.

The professions and their new priorities

In the past, the training of medical professionals equipped them for their role in a cross between a craft industry and a secret society. It focused on making the right intervention in each patient encounter, and allowed them to communicate in abstruse medical language, mainly with other members of the medical priesthood. Of course, this is an exaggeration, but not an enormous one, as reading many of the letters from consultants to referring physicians will demonstrate.

The changes implied by our 10 productivity levers for the medical professions are profound. They will affect their training, their continuing professional development, their use of technology and the mix of tasks they perform. While doctors in training need to study texts and pass exams, later stages focus on learning from direct patient contact under the guidance of their seniors. The assumption is that a doctor needs to recognize and diagnose most of the diseases she is likely to encounter from the hard-wired knowledge in her head, confirming her diagnosis with a range of diagnostic tools, from blood tests to MRI scans. As our biomedical insights continue to fragment traditional diseases into multiple molecular disorders, keeping pace with advance gets tougher and tougher. If certain diseases are encountered rarely, as for example pancreatic cancer in general practice, a potentially fatal disease goes unrecognized. Head knowledge needs increasingly to be complemented by online decision support, distilling the wisdom and experience of the best specialists and putting it at the fingertips (now on the computer screen) of the practitioner.

The system can prompt the doctor to collect the right information to affect the treatment choice and display the overall treatment pathway recommended. In future, the intelligent use of such systems will be valued as highly as the ability to store up clinical knowledge. Continuing Medical Education (CME) must also undergo a revolution. In place of major conferences in distant hotels (enjoyable as these breaks and trips can be) advanced webcast and video tools will carry lectures from world-class specialists, demonstrate procedures, test understanding through interactive case examples, compare alternative treatments, and carry hot news of discoveries and developments.

Progressive doctors are already using IT quite extensively, calling up advice and information from the Web, communicating with their patients by e-mail and text alerts and recording observations and prescriptions electronically. Broadening these habits to the whole profession must be a priority, to create the future 'learning organization'. Technology support will also enable greater use of paramedical technicians in routine procedures, and more use of pharmacists and practice nurses to manage chronic disease, deal with minor ailments, and administer simple treatments. Pharmacists can conduct overall reviews of patients' medication, encourage them to comply and train them in self-management of chronic disease. They bring 'health to the high street' and so into everyday life like no other player in the system.

Collaborative technology will also speed the shift needed from professionals acting in isolation, to being members of a care team for complex cases.

New imperatives for patients, families and communities

For too long patients have seen healthcare as a service into whose hands they fall once disease or trauma strike. It is now time to take charge of our own health destiny.

We should treat our bodies at least as well as we do a new car or any other expensive piece of machinery—with daily care, regular preventative maintenance, and careful attention to early signs of trouble. Huge spending on health magazines, health clubs, and 'nutraceuticals' shows that we desperately want to be healthy and vigorous. But somehow, when it comes to painful action or self-denial to prevent disease occurring, we shut our eyes and hope for the best. Part of the problem lies in our skewed perception of risk and the probability of disease. When we are told: 'you are putting on weight, and not exercising enough—you are at risk for diabetes' it is somehow not quite enough to energize most of us. But in the era of personalized medicine we are entering, it will not be a vague threat we are given, but a defined probability. 'With your genetic profile, and the levels of these specific pre-diabetic proteins in your blood, and with no change to your diet or exercise regime, the chance of diabetes in the next five years is 65 to 75%'. This turns a possibility into a probability – essentially into a pre-diagnosis of disease. Most of us would act on such a prediction.

A Californian company, Tethys, has just such a test now available for diabetes, measuring the level of selected proteins in the blood, and employers are encouraging employees to take the test and then take the action needed to keep them healthy and productive. Tests like this, with the other data captured on our personal health record, will give us the information needed to shoulder more responsibility for our own future. This will be backed up by incentives—in the form of 'carrots' (free health club memberships under our personal health plan) or 'sticks' (large co-payments if we contract an avoidable condition).

A concept being discussed in the UK is a patient-held chronic care budget, placing in the hands of the patient the ability to choose and manage the care they will receive. The main problem is probably that those without the necessary skill or will, and therefore often those most in need, may be least successful in managing long-term budgets. However, such experiments are vital, as they put budgets in the hands of those closest to the real needs—the patients.

Over the 25 years since he left the army, Jane's husband **George** had thickened around the middle. It was a natural part of middle age, he thought, and Jane seemed to agree, as she affectionately pinched his waistline. That was until the doctor, in his annual physical three years ago, calculated his Body Mass Index (BMI), which—at 31—put him in the 'obese' category. But he also measured his metabolic profile using functional MRI and reviewed his genetic profile for predisposition to Type II diabetes. The new proteomic tests confirmed that the risk was a real one, and putting all these results into the latest 'diabetometer' calculation showed that he had a 50% chance of developing the disease in 10 years at current course and speed, but this fell to less than 10% if he adjusted his diet and lost 15 pounds. This finding was enough to convince him to change both diet and exercise habits. He did not even need to see the new simulator that would show him exactly how he would look and feel in 10 years time as a diabetic. His last annual physical showed him on the <10% trajectory as long as he kept up the changes.

While the patient himself has the most at stake, and increasingly the power and incentive to improve his health, he may still not care enough to act. But especially in the case of a man, there is usually a partner that does care. If granted permission, the system could empower partners with the information or disease screening tools they need to overcome the natural, particularly male reluctance to seek help until it is too late.

We must go further and empower the community. This is especially important for immigrant or other ethnic groups, often under-served by the official health system. Community health movements recognize that many of the factors that shape our health come from the communities in which we live. A community's economic prosperity, or lack of it, still has a huge impact. For example, in Britain among the over 50s, people in the poorest fifth of the population have a death rate twice as great for men and nearly four times for women, than found in the top fifth. Health inequalities often mirror income gaps.

Likewise, ethnic groups have very different health profiles, as a result of diet, lifestyle, and genetics. People from the Indian sub-continent, even when living in the UK or US, have a diet higher in fats and suffer from higher levels of diabetes than others in the same geographical areas. In the UK, men born in South Asia are 50% more likely to have angina or heart attacks. In a disadvantaged part of East London, a charity supported by a major pharmaceutical company helps a South Asian community at heightened risk of diabetes and heart disease spot the early signs and get help. We must not allow misplaced political correctness (a policy blind spot in Britain) to prevent us from designing community health programmes to meet specific ethnic needs.

Access to the health system is another key factor. Many communities do not have sufficient general practitioners from their ethnic groups, and some come from a culture in which GPs are not consulted and all ailments are taken directly to hospital, often too late. This is particularly true of many in the

African-American and Latino populations in the US, a trend reinforced in the past by lower levels of health insurance.

A community's detachment from the system, their diet and the lack of general practitioners speaking the right language, can easily combine to create or worsen problems. Media channels, places, and people designed to reach these communities can literally be life-lines, and deserve official funding. Education has an impact on how aware people are of their own health risks and options. This makes a new form of prescription of critical importance—the 'information prescription'. Alongside whatever treatment or drug prescription we receive from a visit to the doctor, we should receive our 'information prescription', containing information on the disease, treatment options, and actions we ourselves can take to speed recovery. These prescriptions, in the right simple language matched to the person and situation, will help each of us take the responsibility we must, if our own care is to be effective and affordable.

Chapter 5

Conclusion—the US, the UK, and the Middle Way

Few challenges we face are as far-reaching as the quality and sustainability of our health care. Health, or lack of it, reaches into every corner of our lives— our self-esteem and confidence, our employability, the coherence of our families, our household finances, and our view of the future. So it is not surprising that health system problems often dominate political campaigns. If we follow the trends in supply and demand, in technology and expectations, in costs of care and shifts in population, it is easy to be pessimistic. Each generation of politicians will hope that the meltdown forecast in this book won't happen 'on their watch'. But look around—the early signs are already there, in the sheer level of spending and the rising tide of dissatisfaction with what we get for it.

Very different models—markets versus management

Where to look for the best approach to the problem—the UK or the US? 3000 miles: when it comes to healthcare, the UK and the US could not be further apart. The UK looks at the US and sees runaway costs, private profiteering, and over 40 million uninsured. The US looks at the UK and sees socialized medicine, rundown facilities, rationing of treatment, and 'death panels'.

Of course, viable solutions for sustainable health systems will inevitably be shaped by the values of the society in which they sit. Any system in the US, even one mandated by the Federal Government, will reflect American emphasis on individuality and choice. As a result of this demand for choice and of employment mobility, US private health plans will still be subject to periodic membership switching, making long-term health returns more difficult to capture. *multiple comments about this*

Healthcare reform in the US, now finally arrived, is in practice just healthcare *insurance* reform. The fragmentation of the US 'system', on both the payer and provider sides, makes any comprehensive reform of how care is delivered a virtually impossible task.

Funding healthcare through central taxation, the UK model, creates the maximum size of risk pool, but it separates responsibility for raising money from that for spending it. It also makes the total budget vulnerable to swings in the national economy and public sector deficit.

Restructuring or reforming the NHS also faces major cultural obstacles. Ever since its creation, both people and politicians have seen the NHS as a state-provided system of doctors and hospitals to which they are entitled, rather than as a health insurance plan that delivers benefits in proportion to public funding. This has led to the absurdity of a centrally-managed organization of 1.2 million people, with 'managers' seeking to direct professionals who are often loyal to their interest groups and their own notions of what the NHS stands for, rather than to the patient care units of which they are part.

With the urgent need to tackle an impeding medical meltdown in both the US and UK systems, perhaps we should ask the question: is there a Middle Way, a 'mid-Atlantic' solution? One that combines the best of wise management and free markets?

Markets or Management—which is the best prescription for healthcare?

The US health system is an open market in many respects. Doctors, hospitals, provider systems, and health insurance plans all compete with their peers, and many of the prices they charge are theirs to set, to reflect value and attract customers.

The UK system is heavily managed, with very limited market mechanisms. Central government allocates budgets, sets salaries (by negotiation with professional bodies), issues guidelines and targets and appoints management. It also sets national reimbursement rates and agrees drug prices. There is some competition (rendered more politically acceptable by the label 'contestability'), but this tends to be at the margin, to meet needs in underserved areas. Introducing competitors to the 'official' system is predictably unpopular with state employees and with professional bodies like the British Medical Association.

Both approaches—top-down management and free market mechanisms—are controversial. Markets squeeze out those who cannot afford the prices they set. Command-and-control management quenches initiative and forgoes the efficiency benefits that come from competition.

In fact, the ideal healthcare system needs a mix of markets and management, since both bring benefits the other cannot.

Markets are good at balancing supply and demand, at least over the longer term, and at setting efficient prices as a result. They are more responsive to the demands of customers who have choice, and better at releasing the energy and initiative of competing firms and employees. Excellence is more likely except where competition is weak or customers undemanding.

(Continued)

Management is good at setting consistent standards and requiring reporting against them. It optimizes the allocation of resources. While it may not be effective at creating IT and other infrastructure, it can effectively mandate its use.

In a Middle Way, central management would play a very defined role in setting minimum standards for access, outcomes, and finance and requiring consistent reporting against them, so that patients can make informed choices. It would insist (e.g. by making this a condition of payment) on the use of interoperable information systems, so that professionals or patients see fewer barriers to moving between different providers. It would tilt the playing field in favour of integrated health systems in other ways also, insisting on commissioning bids for total population coverage and provision.

However, all of the rest of the system would be shaped mainly by open competition—including salaries, prices, incentives, management approaches, organizational structures, and capital investments. Subject, of course, to regulation to prevent abuses.

Moving towards the right mix for the UK is politically very sensitive, because of the long-held belief that the NHS stands for absolute consistency and predictability, whoever you are and wherever you live. No market-driven provision system can guarantee this, but what it can guarantee is greater efficiency in the use of resources and greater responsiveness to customer need.

Bringing any central management into the US would be no less controversial, as the fierce responses to 'health reform' initiatives consistently show. However, setting rules on comprehensive coverage without 'preexisting condition' penalties, mandating interoperable EMR systems, constraining medical liability awards, and insisting on consistent reporting against access, financial and outcome standards—these would shape the landscape for efficient competition.

The result of moving towards the centre will not be a UK system that looks and feels like the US, but one that takes advantage of competition to drive performance. The result for the US would be far from 'socialized medicine' but it would create a system where fairness and productivity is wired in, without choice being restricted.

Without such changes, both systems face the risk of unaffordable healthcare, but for different reasons and at different rates. The US is likely to experience more consumer- and provider-driven demand growth and will want to afford as much new technology as possible. With ObamaCare offering universal coverage, private sector insurers and profit-centred doctors and hospitals look likely to continue to drive up health insurance premiums and deductibles. Government will be tempted to step in to control them.

The UK will still be tempted to cap the money available to the NHS irrespective of its economic contribution, to try to run its giant organization from the centre, and deal with the gap between budgets and patient demands by issuing guidelines and edicts that ration access to care or new technology. It is vital that these temptations are resisted, and early indications from the 2010 Coalition Government are encouraging.

So far, discussion between policymakers on each side of the Atlantic has been largely a dialogue of the deaf. Admittedly, from time to time there has been a desire in the UK to learn from some of the more rational integrated US systems, notably Kaiser Permanente. And the US has studied and considered importing management tools from the UK, notably the National Institute for Clinical Excellence. But largely each side has looked across the Atlantic and told themselves: 'our system may have its problems, but at least we don't have theirs!'

It is time to see if a Middle Way might work better for both.

Learning from the best—and worst—of both

What are the best practice principles, or warnings, from each that could enable us to construct a Middle Way?

From the US experience we learn, among other things, that:

- Government need not run the system, but does need to set the ground rules and define success if the whole population is to benefit
- Healthcare providers can run as profitable businesses and still deliver high quality care
- Hospital emergency rooms are a very inefficient way to deal with minor ailments or preventable problems
- Choice between health plans can drive competition for cost-effectiveness in commissioning
- Medical innovation can spread outwards from major medical centres as 'innovation hubs', investing heavily in research alongside routine care
- Integrated health systems work better than fragmented primary and secondary care providers.

From the UK we learn, among other things, that:

- Universal coverage is affordable
- Insistence on value can influence clinical behaviour, but crude rationing based on a 'fixed pot' is highly unpopular
- A culture of service to patients and the community can be a driving principle in dedicated delivery of care
- Central management of the system quenches local professional initiative and produces unintended consequences
- Insistence on equality can trump quality.

The key features of the two systems are compared in Figure 5.1.

Figure 5.1 Healthcare systems - UK and US comparison

		UK	US
Features	Public vs private funding	90:10	50:50
	Choice of health plan	One–NHS	Multiple plans
	Patient co-funding of care	Free at point of need	Varies with plan
	Access to specialists	Controlled by GP	Direct if 'in plan'
	Access to medicines	National & local control	Little/no direct control
	Provider competition	Limited competition	Free competition
	Provider management	Top-down national mgt	Only within IHS systems
	Integration of care	Theoretically, via GP	Only in IHS systems
	Strengths	Universal coverage	Islands of excellence
		Overall budget control	Patient choice
	Weaknesses	Top-down management	40+ million uninsured
		Limited choice	High total bill
		Little competition	Costly defensive medicine
		Low access to innovation	

Neither formula leads to outstanding results: both have among the highest levels of 'mortality amenable to healthcare'—deaths that good healthcare could have prevented. Most European countries have 60–90 such deaths per 100,000, while both the UK and the US are above 100.

It is not lack of regulation or guidance that holds back the NHS—it is the sheer weight of it (see Figure 5.2). As the system developed, layer on layer of bodies to guide decisions have been added. It is no surprise that initiative and entrepreneurism have suffered.

A Middle Way?

A Middle Way that both systems should move towards would have the following features:

- A role for government that ensures universal coverage at acceptable minimum standards and affordable cost, but does not seek to manage healthcare delivery
- Competitive health plans that commission for value, measured in terms of quality of care, acceptable costs of delivering it, and speedy access and positive experience for patients
- Management and regulation of providers that provides the right financial incentives to be innovative and productive, monitors performance, shares best practice, and tracks outcomes
- *Patients that are well-informed about the choices open to them and actively engaged in managing their own health, with the support of their communities.*

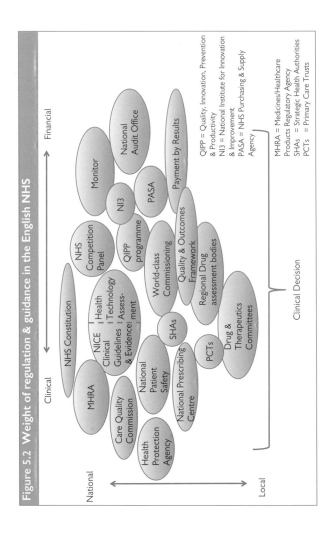

Figure 5.2 Weight of regulation & guidance in the English NHS

Clinical — Financial

National — Local

- NHS Constitution
- MHRA
- Care Quality Commission
- Health Protection Agency
- National Patient Safety
- National Prescribing Centre
- NICE Clinical Guidelines & Evidence
- Health Technology Assessment
- SHAs
- PCTs
- Drug & Therapeutics Committees
- NHS Competition Panel
- QIPP programme
- World-class Commissioning
- Quality & Outcomes Framework
- Regional Drug assessment bodies
- Monitor
- NI3
- PASA
- National Audit Office
- Payment by Results

Clinical Decision

QIPP = Quality, Innovation, Prevention & Productivity
NI3 = National Institute for Innovation & Improvement
PASA = NHS Purchasing & Supply Agency

MHRA = Medicines/Healthcare Products Regulatory Agency
SHAs = Strategic Health Authorities
PCTs = Primary Care Trusts

It is time for the US to lose its paranoia about 'socialized medicine' and recognize that a 21st century society without quality care for all is indefensible. It is time for the UK to lose its fond attachment to the idea of the NHS as a perfect system spoiled only by imperfect people.

It is also the right time for those building new health systems in the fast-developing countries such as China, India, and Brazil to learn the lessons from both the market-driven and management-dominated approaches, and to create the right mix for their cultures.

For healthcare can and must combine the best of both, using the levers laid out in this book. Or the future of medicine will fail the test of sustainability.

If we fail to rise to the challenge of sustainable healthcare, the 'Carters', that is our own children and grandchildren, will not easily forgive us.

Epilogue

This short book cannot do more than scratch the surface of the debate we need to have on the future of medicine and healthcare. Therefore we have set up a website *www.2030Healthfutures.com* for readers to share their views on the challenges and proposals for healthcare in 2030.

Further reading

Clayton M Christiensen, with Jerome Grossman and Jason Hwang, *The Innovator's Prescription*, McGraw Hill (2009)

Tom Daschle, with Scott E Greenberger and Jeanne M Lambrew, *Critical – What we can do about the health-care crisis*, Thomas Dunne Books (2008)

James Le Fanu, *The Rise and Fall of Modern Medicine*, Abacus (1999)

Daniel Kahnemann, *QALYs versus Experience: A perspective from experimental economics*, Office of Health Economics (2007)

Bill Moyes and Paul Corrigan, *Future Foundations—Towards a new culture in the NHS*, Policy Exchange (2010)

Michael E Porter and Elizabeth Olmsted Teisberg, *Redefining Health Care*, Harvard Business School Press (2006)

Matt Ridley, *Genome*, Harper Collins (1999)

Index

Note: page numbers in *italics* refer to Figures.